A Guide to Independence for the Visually Impaired and Their Families

by

Vivian Younger and Jill Sardegna

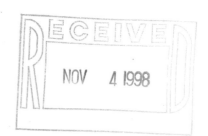

Demos Publications, 386 Park Avenue South, New York, New York 10016

Library of Congress Cataloging-in-Publication Data
Younger, Vivian.
   A guide to independence for the visually impaired and their families / by Vivian Younger and Jill Sardegna.
       p.   cm.
   Includes bibliographical references and index.
   ISBN 0-939957-61-2
   1. Visually handicapped—United States—Life skills and guides.
2. Blind—United States—Life skills guides.   I. Sardegna, Jill.
II. Title.
HV1795.Y68   1994
362.4'1—dc20   94-26012
                                                      CIP

Dedication

*To Peggy Dodge and
the Braille Transcription Project of Santa
Clara County,
Norman and Nadia Kaplan,
and Mary Ellen Rogers*

*To Deborah Gilden, Harry Murphy, and
Carol Ranalli*

About the Authors

VIVIAN YOUNGER is a generalist vocational counselor for the California State Department of Rehabilitation in San Jose, California. Although she now counsels people of all disabilities, she has specialized in working with the blind as a teacher/counselor.

Younger has experienced a progressive sight loss all her life. She is an active member of the disabled community and has served on the Santa Clara County Commission on the Status of Women, the Disability Advisory Committee for the City of San Jose, the Santa Clara County Commission for the Developmentally Disabled, and the Board of Directors for the Santa Clara County Blind Center. Younger was co-chairwoman for the Conference for Women with Disabilities for four years and was the recipient of the Santa Clara County Woman of Achievement Award for 1980.

Younger is the former director of the "Take A Giant Step" (TAGS) program, a recreation, education, and social program for visually impaired children, and has presented seminars on disabilities and Black history.

During her college years, Younger was honored as a Dean's Scholar and was selected for inclusion in "Who's Who Among Students in American Universities and Colleges." She holds a B.A. degree in Liberal Studies and an M.A. degree in Public Administration. Younger lives in San Jose.

JILL SARDEGNA is a freelance writer and author of the books *The Encyclopedia of Blindness and Vision Impairment* and *K Is for Kiss Good Night*.

Sardegna is also a playwright. Her two-act play, *Specs*, features a blind protagonist and was chosen by the Disabled Students Theatre Group of California State University at Northridge for production in June 1990.

Sardegna is a former teacher and exhibit developer for the Children's Discovery Museum of San Jose, where she developed the traveling exhibit "One Way or Another," a hands-on exhibit designed to teach children about disabilities. She has served as the Materials Director for the Conference for Women with Disabilities and written articles about disabilities and children's fears concerning disabilities.

Sardegna received her B.A. degree in Liberal Studies and her M.A. degree in Instructional Technology. She lives in San Jose with her husband and daughter.

Acknowledgments

We want to offer our appreciation to the following individuals for their contributions to this book: Dr. Peter D'Alena, Norman Kaplan, Dr. Edwin B. Mehr, Dr. Harry J. Murphy, Carol A. Ranalli, The Braille Transcription Project of Santa Clara County, Inc., and our anonymous friends who supplied us with personal Journal Notes. Our special thanks to Dr. Deborah Gilden for her exhaustive and thorough counsel, guidance, and advice.

Vivian Younger
Jill Sardegna
San Jose, CA, 1994

Contents

How To Use This Book

This guide is a hands-on approach to helping you, your family, and your friends now that you are losing your sight. Its goal is to help you become more independent and to help family members and friends who want to be supportive but do not know how. This book will teach you how to perform basic tasks of daily living, how to address new and puzzling feelings and fears, how to respond to embarrassing situations, how to appropriately assess behavior and stages of growth, and how to find additional help and information regarding sight loss.

This book can serve as a supplement to formal rehabilitation programs or as an alternative source of information for those of you who choose not to seek such formal training. It is not a substitute for formal rehabilitation programs. It does provide some instructions taught in such programs, but only those that require no formal training to teach.

The guide is written in a nontechnical, basic style that allows it to present task instructions in a step-by-step manner. Some of the instructions may seem simplistic or obvious to you because we describe them in such detail. If this is the case, ignore the obvious and make use of the information appropriate for your needs. Our intention is to provide information that will meet a wide range of needs for those with low vision and those with no vision. Since each chapter was designed to be used independent of the others, you can take what you need from one, several, or all chapters, as you need it.

There are many terms to describe vision loss, including *visually impaired*, *visually handicapped*, *visually limited*, and *visually disabled*. We use the term *visually impaired* with the understanding that vision can vary greatly from individual to individual. We reserve the word *blind* for those who have no light perception.

We accept the American Foundation for the Blind's definitions of *low vision* and *legal blindness*. A person with low vision is defined as having a visual acuity of 20/50 in the better eye, with correction, or a visual field of 40 to 20 degrees or less. The term *legally blind* is a description of vision loss that the government uses to determine eligibility for governmental assistance. A legally blind person is defined as one who has 20/200 visual acuity in the better eye with correction, or a field of vision of equal to or less than 20 degrees.

These terms are confusing, so here are some brief definitions. The term *visual acuity* describes the distance a person can see compared to the distance that a person with normal vision can see. In other words, if you can see at twenty feet what a person with normal vision can see at twenty feet, your visual acuity is 20/20. If you see at twenty feet what a person with normal vision sees at two hundred feet, your visual acuity is 20/200.

> **Journal Note:** I am legally blind. I see 20/200. My vision ability is much like an out-of-focus projector. I am able to see color. I am able to read standard print at about half a page at a time. I am self-employed as a small engine technician/mechanic. I work on lawn mowers, steam cleaners, etc. When reading technical manuals, microfiche, catalogs, and when I do detailed work, I use the equivalent of a jeweler's lens extension.
> —*Louis*

The *visual field* is the measurement of area you can see. It is measured by degrees, with 180 degrees as the normal standard. You may have a loss of central vision, a loss of the middle part of the visual field, or a loss of peripheral vision (the side sections of the visual field). Some people even have "branches" of vision loss at various places in the visual field.

Vision loss or blindness may be either *congenital* or *adventitious*. Congenital blindness or vision loss is present at birth or shortly afterward. Adventitious vision loss or blindness occurs after five years of age as a result of a disease or an injury to the eye.

> **Journal Note:** I am seventy years old. I lost my vision eight years ago following a routine physical and eye exam. I found out that I had glaucoma. In order to prevent my optic nerve from further deterioration, surgery was recommended and immediately performed. Five surgeries later, I am able to see large print, colors, standard print (enough to read one or two words or a phone number) and see objects depending on environmental conditions such as lighting, color, and contrast.
>
> *—Rose*

Although visually impaired persons may retain some usable vision, its level may fluctuate significantly. This may lead to misunderstandings because the family may suspect that their loved one is faking or lying about their vision. The visually impaired person can help the family understand his or her vision loss by explaining, in detail, how much vision he or she has and how it fluctuates.

> **Journal Note:** When a person has low vision and their vision changes from day to day, it is sometimes hard to convey unfamiliar vision experiences. For example, I periodically see a white cloud over my eyes for one to two minutes.
>
> *—Julia*

> **Journal Note:** I have retinitis pigmentosa. During the day I can see large objects, such as trees, buildings, and

lawns, but I am totally blind at night. I use my residual vision and long white cane for safe traveling. I occasionally say "hello" to posts.

—John

Those with central vision loss, which occurs in conditions such as age-related maculopathy (macular degeneration), may lose the vision in the middle of their visual field but retain some peripheral vision. Although they may not be able to see their dinner plate, their remaining side (peripheral) vision may allow them to see the water glass or silverware alongside it.

Those with diabetic retinopathy may experience a blurring in the central field of vision. Cataracts may cause a general blurring of the entire field, somewhat like looking through waxed paper. People with a detached retina or other visual conditions resulting from a disease or medical condition, such as multiple sclerosis, lupus, or stroke, may experience double vision, uncontrollable eye movements, or they may view the world around blocked areas of vision, an effect similar to that of looking through tree branches.

Those with a peripheral vision loss caused by glaucoma, retinitis pigmentosa (RP), and other conditions may have tunnel vision and view life as if they were looking through a straw. Others may only be able to distinguish between light and shadow.

> **Journal Note:** I lost my sight gradually due to a detached retina. I currently can see light, dark, and occasional shadows. I am one of five brothers who are blind in my family.
>
> *—Michael*

Consult Your Physician

These descriptions and others found in this book are not intended as diagnostic tools. We urge you to ask your doctor or ophthalmologist for information relating to your or your loved one's individual circumstances. We urge you to get your doctor's or ophthalmologist's advice and consent before undergoing any rehabilitation program or activity suggested in this book.

Which doctor or specialist should you consult? At one point or another, you may consult an ophthalmologist, an optometrist, a low vision specialist, an optician, a rehabilitation counselor, a special education teacher, or an orientation and mobility instructor. Each specialist is responsible for a different portion of your treatment or therapeutic program.

An *ophthalmologist* is a medical doctor who has completed specialized residency training in diseases and surgery of the eye. Many ophthalmologists receive additional training in subspecialties, such as cornea transplant surgery, retinal surgery, or low vision services. Ophthalmologists test vision, prescribe corrective lenses, diagnose and treat eye diseases and defects, prescribe medications, and perform surgery.

An *optometrist* holds a degree in optometry, which is awarded after completing college and four years of optometry school. Optometrists screen and diagnose common eye problems, assess the efficiency and health of the eyes, prescribe and dispense corrective eyeglasses and contact lenses. Optometrists are not physicians; they refer patients to a physician or an ophthalmologist when disease is present or surgery is indicated.

An *optician* dispenses the lenses and low vision aids prescribed by ophthalmologists and optometrists. Opticians grind and formulate lenses and fit them to a frame. In many states, opticians also fit and administer contact lenses. They are not trained or licensed to examine the eyes or to prescribe lenses.

Most *low vision specialists* are optometrists who perform the low vision clinical examination, analyze and evaluate the information, and prescribe low vision aids. Assessment information may be obtained and evaluated by them, while training may be provided by other professionals, such as social workers, educators, occupational therapists, counselors, rehabilitation instructors, vocational counselors for the blind, and orientation and mobility specialists.

Rehabilitation instructors are trained and experienced in working with people who have disabilities. They provide assessment and goal setting services, teach daily living and organization skills, and provide prevocational and vocational training. (See Chapter 12.) *Orientation and mobility instructors* teach visually impaired people how to travel safely and independently. This type of training may include instruction in the use of a long white cane or electronic and optical traveling aids.

Dear Diary

You will find Journal Notes sprinkled throughout the text. These are the personal experiences of the authors, their friends, and their colleagues. They express the gamut of feelings—from pain to humor—that visually impaired people and their families may experience, and offer some unique ways of dealing with awkward situations.

Finally, we have written in a lighthearted, humorous tone. This is not intended to trivialize the trauma of losing your sight, but rather to lift your spirits and encourage you to learn how to cope with blindness in a positive way. We maintain a positive outlook because we truly believe that you can do almost anything.

2

Initial Reactions to Vision Loss

Just as there are many causes of loss of sight, there are many reactions that you may have to your vision loss. Your personality, past experiences with blindness, education, social and financial factors, mobility, occupation, cultural background, general physical condition, psychological readiness (motivation), and family support system will all affect how you deal with your vision loss.

Most people are devastated when they learn that they are losing their vision or will become legally blind. And little wonder! The fear of darkness (often equated with blindness) is often among the most common fears people have. Blindness is so feared, in fact, that other more potentially dangerous diseases may be perceived as less threatening and more welcome than visual impairment.

The first reaction to a diagnosis of vision loss is usually a mixture of shock, fear, and confusion. You may be afraid that you will not be able to function independently. You may feel loss of self-identity and resistance to thinking of yourself as "one of those blind people." You might also question whether your doctor has made an accurate diagnosis.

In her book *On Death and Dying*, Dr. Elisabeth Kubler-Ross describes the five emotional stages that accompany a death or loss: denial, anger, bargaining, depression, and acceptance. You may find yourself going through some of the same stages during your experience of vision loss.

The Process of Denial

Kubler-Ross describes denial as a temporary defense. You may want to think of it as "The Great Stall." After all, if you don't think about your vision loss, you don't have to deal with it, right?

Denial can take many forms. You may refuse to admit that you have a vision loss. You may decline to talk about your sight loss and avoid people who want to talk about it. You may refuse to wear your glasses or hold onto a friend's arm, even when it is common sense to do so. You even may go so far as to walk into a post in your need to deny your vision loss!

As you rub your aching nose, you may come to the realization that your lack of vision cannot be ignored. Although some people successfully deny vision loss for great periods of time, life has a way of setting up posts in the most unexpected places.

If you have reached such a roadblock but find talking about your vision loss too painful, try just thinking about the problem. You may be able to deal with this for only five-minute periods at first. Look at this as progress. Accept the fact that most people feel the need to deny their problems at one time or another. Even when you have moved on to another stage of the grieving process, you may find yourself reverting to denial occasionally.

> **Journal Note:** I denied my legal blindness for years. In order to continue driving, I would ask a family member to point out landmarks and which lane to turn into. Although I hit someone on a bike (fortunately, this person was not seriously hurt), I continued to drive. Losing independence and the privilege to drive was emotionally painful to me. It was not until I was in a car accident that I was forced to face my overdue vision denial.
>
> —*Pam*

As a friend or relative, you can help your loved one by being open to discussing the challenge of vision loss. But don't push. Allow him to have his defenses for now. Trust that there is a post out there somewhere with his name on it.

All the Rage

Once you have acknowledged that you have a vision loss, anger may set in. With good reason, you may think, "Why me?" Indeed, why you? Those around you with normal vision may infuriate you since they remind you of what you have lost. You may feel that they take their vision for granted. Even though you know it is uncharitable and wish them no harm, you may still be left feeling, "Why me? Why not them?"

You may also resist participating in sight-related activities. "Why should I watch TV—I can't see it anyway," you may think. This is also part of your anger. Vision-oriented activities remind you what it was like to be able to see and point out how painful the loss of sight is to you. Unfortunately, at first, you may find something that makes you angry everywhere you look.

Those around you may also treat you differently. Friends or relatives may insist on doing even the most simple chores for you, from opening doors to tying your shoes—no wonder you feel helpless. They may have gotten into the habit of talking about you as if you are not present—no wonder you feel invisible. They may even have gone so far as to assume that since you are losing your sight, you are also losing your mind, and try to make all your decisions for you—no wonder you feel angry.

> **Journal Note:** It makes me angry when someone assumes that I lack intelligence because I'm blind. As if the state of my eyes is directly related to the state of my mind. But because this is a sore point with me, I have to be careful that I don't assume things myself. Once in a candy store, I asked the saleswoman to describe some Christmas candy shapes to me. She sounded exasperated and treated me as though I had limited intelligence. As I started to boil over, another customer spoke up and said, "I don't think this sales lady realizes you have a vision problem." Whoops, I assumed she was reacting badly to my blindness, when she just had a negative attitude in general.   *Vivian*

Your anger may reach frightening proportions if you have always been a very independent person. You may greet any assistance or sympathy with rage, and you may hate your perceived dependence on others so much that you feel that you want to strike out and hit something or someone. Well, that is what punching bags were invented for. If you do not happen to have a punching bag handy, punch your pillow. Have an old-fashioned pillow fight, kick the bed, or lay down on the floor and scream. Go ahead. Who's to know? You have a right to be angry and you will feel better once your feelings are out in the open.

After you calm down, you may notice that you are displacing some of your anger onto friends, relatives, or doctors. You may find yourself thinking, "If that doctor were any good, he would have prevented this." You may have shouted at your daughter, "Why can't you make the coffee right? Your help is worse than none at all!" You may feel resentful of the help of others and intolerant of their pity, but try to remember that your vision problem is not their fault. Sometimes just saying (or even shouting), "I'm sorry. I'm not angry at you. I'm just angry," will help them understand. Remember that they are experiencing their own reactions to your vision loss.

As a friend or relative, try not to take this anger personally. Remember that you, with your vision, are a constant reminder of what your loved one has lost. You will go on enjoying things in ways he or she no longer can. Although his or her reactions may be demanding, infuriating, and inappropriate, your emotional support is greatly needed. This may be difficult for you, and you may want to indulge in a bit of pillow-bashing yourself.

Let's Make a Deal

The third stage in the grieving process is bargaining. During this stage you may try to make deals with God, the Fates, or any higher being you hold dear. You may find yourself saying, "If only I could see again, I would devote my life to the blind," or "If I got my sight back, I would never take it for granted again." These are worthy wishes and if for any reason your sight should return, it would probably benefit you to follow up on these projects. However, since life often turns out to be the better negotiator, these deals frequently fall through.

> **Journal Note:** When I first started to lose my sight, I felt very depressed. I often asked God, "Why me?" and often felt that God was punishing me for something that I didn't do. I would say to God, "If I had my sight, I would make a better life for myself." After seven years of being blind, I see blindness as a nuisance, not a handicap. I feel now that there isn't enough time in the day to do all the things I want to do in my life.
>
> *—Michael*

Desolation Valley

During the fourth stage of the grieving process—depression—feelings of loss begin to replace your anger. You may lose your appetite, feel a loss of energy, or lose interest in activities around you. You may feel as though you are just going through the motions of each day. Because you do not yet know how to adapt to the sighted world, you may feel isolated from yourself and from others. Questions such as "Who am I?" and "What will become of me?" may run through your mind.

The more isolated you become, the more lonely, different, and cast-out you may feel. You may have trouble expressing your feelings. The anger that once easily found expression in everything you said may now be replaced by feelings of hopelessness and despair that are unable to find an outlet.

> **Journal Note:** When I was informed that I was legally blind and that my eye condition was progressive, I felt devastated. At first, I blamed everyone for my vision

loss. At times, I felt very depressed and was unsure about what was in store for me. I worried about losing my job and whether my company would be able to train me in another department. At times I felt so alone. Although my family members were supportive I don't think they really understood what it is like to see your vision fading away. They don't understand that I may start bumping into certain objects because I've lost more vision. Well, it took me two and one half years to accept that I was going to be visually impaired for the rest of my life.

—Susan

It is important to take steps that will make you feel less iso-lated. Talk to a trusted friend or relative. Don't be afraid that you will sound self-pitying—you need to share these feelings with someone. "Hey, I need to talk for a minute, okay?" may be all you need to say.

It is also helpful to read about or meet others who have expe-rienced similar types and degrees of vision loss. Call your local library or the National Library Service for the Blind and Physically Handicapped (800-424-9100) and ask them to recommend some books about blindness or about people who have experienced a vision loss. Ask a friend or relative to read the books to you, or check with the librarian about books on cassette tape or volunteer agencies that can tape them for you. This task is not to inspire you to become the "World Champion Blind Person." It is just to provide you with an avenue to share the same feelings, pain, and success that others have gone through.

No matter how strong your character or how supportive your family, you may still feel lost sometimes. If this is the case, you may want to seek professional help. Consider discussing your feel-ings with your doctor, a counselor, a therapist, your clergyman, a referral hot line operator, or a volunteer for an organization for the blind. You may want to talk with one or more of these people.

The important thing is not to give up if your first few attempts do not bring the relief you seek. Keep calling and trying until you get the help you need.

Try not to feel rejected if some potential supporters can not help you immediately. They may ask you to call back in a few weeks or ask you to schedule your first meeting for as much as a month later. Even though such delays are normal, in your present emotional state you may feel rejected.

> **Journal Note:** I am blind as a result of retinitis pigmentosa. I lost my sight gradually. I think that gradually losing my sight helped me to adjust slowly to my blindness.
>
> —*Frank*

Accept the Consequences

As you begin to function without your sight or with limited vision, you will come closer and closer to acceptance. Throughout this period you will experience joy, pain, disappointment, surprise, fear, and laughter—the whole spectrum of emotions. Keep in mind that acceptance is a relative thing. Long after you reach some level of acceptance, you will still have moments of resentment and anger.

> **Journal Note:** I became legally blind at age 17 due to a form of multiple sclerosis. I had partial vision up until I was 27 years old. I just woke up one day totally blind. It took my brother much more time to accept my vision loss than it took me. Occasionally I feel very angry, frustrated, and depressed about being blind. Since I'm the kind of person who wants to make the best of my life, these down moments are rare.
>
> —*Rachael*

Journal Note: I've accepted my blindness but I haven't accepted the limitations imposed by it. I love going to movies and accept that I won't see all the action, but I still feel cheated when everyone laughs at a visual joke and I'm left wondering, "What happened?" As a "worst case" in this situation, I just make up my own scenario.

—Vivian

By now you may be thinking, "Do I have to be happy about being blind to fully accept my blindness?" The answer is no. Accepting your vision loss does not necessarily mean delighting in it. Although you may never be happy about being blind, you still can be a happy person.

Journal Note: I imagine it is very difficult to lose your sight very suddenly. Although I will eventually be totally blind, I'm glad I have the opportunity to hold onto my sight for as long as possible. I treasure every moment that I can see. I think the most important thing about losing your sight is that you have friends and blind role models to talk to.

—Susan

When you are ready to pursue knowledge about blindness and share your feelings about your vision condition, you will be showing signs of acceptance. You may be thinking about learning to read braille or large print, or you may have an interest in devices that can help improve or enhance the vision you now have. You may even be thinking about resuming activities that you abandoned just a short time ago. These are indications that you are beginning to accept your vision loss and are now ready to live your life more fully.

Organizational Checklist

- Talk to a friend or relative about your feelings and concerns regarding your visual impairment.
- Call your local library and ask about books on blindness or about people who have had a vision loss.
- Ask the librarian about books on tape and agencies that tape books for the visually impaired and the general public.
- Seek professional help if needed.

3

Things You Can Do Now

When you were first told you were losing your vision, you may have been so shocked that you were not able to absorb any other information your doctor gave you. In order to help you move through the stages toward acceptance, you need to know exactly what you are dealing with. What caused your vision loss? Can you expect it to get better or worse? How many other people have this eye condition? To obtain the answers to these and other questions, start by talking to your doctor.

When you make an appointment for a consultation, stress that you have many questions about your eye condition and that you will need extra time to have them answered. Add that you would like copies of any brochures your doctor has about your eye disease. This will give him a chance to prepare for your visit.

A Questionable Method

To make the best use of this consultation, you also should do some homework. Make a list of questions to take with you. If you cannot write, record them on a cassette tape. Do not try to do this the day before the visit. Start as soon as you make the appointment and add new questions as they occur to you. Some sample questions follow:

What is wrong with my eyes?

Why don't they work? What caused this vision loss?

What is the name of my eye disease or condition? Please spell it.

How many other people with this condition do you treat each year?

What is the prognosis? Will it get better, worse, or stay the same?

If it gets worse, how much vision can I expect to have in one year? In five years? In ten years?

If my visual condition can improve, what can I do to help it along?

What treatment plan do you have in mind for me?

Will I need to take any medications? If so, please spell them.

How often are they taken? Are they taken with food? With milk?

Do these medications have any side effects?

Will I need eye surgery? If so, please describe the procedure.

Are there any complications to the surgery?

Will any procedures, such as laser treatments, be necessary? If so, please describe these procedures.

Will I need to wear special lenses?

What can I do to preserve or enhance the sight I have?

Should I wear protective lenses or sunglasses in sunlight?

Should I restrict any activities such as lifting heavy objects or bending over?

Is there something I can change in my diet, environment, exercise, or rest schedule to help my eye condition?

Will my vision change at certain times of the day or in different lighting conditions? Will I experience night blindness?

Will my eyes take longer to adapt to changes in light and dark?

Would the use of color or light and dark contrast inside and outside my home help my vision?

Are there adaptive optical or nonoptical aids I can use? Where can I buy them?

What is the latest research on my eye condition?

Where can I go to get more information about my visual impairment?

What are the names of organizations for the visually impaired? How can I contact them?

What books about my type of vision loss would you recommend?

Do you know a person (patient or professional) who has gone through an experience similar to mine? May I contact him or her?

Should I go through any rehabilitation or training programs? If so, what is available?

Where can I go to participate in educational or recreational programs for people with similar vision conditions?

Can you give me a written certification of the degree of visual impairment I have so that I can take advantage of services or programs for the visually impaired?

Do you know if I am eligible for any financial aid as a result of my visual impairment?

If you have made your list of questions on tape, you may want to ask a friend to transfer it to paper both for reinforcement and for the sake of expediency. Some people find it helpful to have the support of a friend or relative during this visit to the eye doctor. Take a blank tape and cassette recorder with you to the appointment in order to tape the doctor's replies for later review. Ask the doctor's permission to tape his responses before you start to record. If you want to attend the appointment alone, you might want to take two cassette recorders—one to play the questions and one to record the answers.

Your Attitude Toward Doctors

Take a moment to get in touch with your general attitude toward doctors. This is important because your viewpoint affects how you approach your health care. You may see doctors as friends, gods, quacks, miracle workers, or final authorities, among other things. If you tend to see doctors as all-knowing, you may be intimidated about questioning a medication or procedure. If you see them as know-nothings, you may be unwilling to accept the appropriate care they prescribe. Try to view your doctor as a *partner* in the care and preservation of your vision. If, after careful thought, you find the partnership less than equal, you may wish to find a new doctor.

> **Journal Note:** I have experienced frustration and dissatisfaction with eye doctors I've seen. One doctor refused to answer any of my questions. Needless to say, we had a short doctor-patient relationship.
> —*Julia*

Doctors occasionally disclose information to you according to your willingness to accept it. If your doctor suspects that you cannot or will not be able to deal with an unsettling diagnosis, he or she may initially be hesitant to give you the full prognosis.

> **Journal Note:** I have seen many eye doctors in my lifetime. Many of them were not willing to share information regarding my eye condition. They seemed hesi-

tant to answer many of my questions. I think they were overprotective and had reservations about my being able to handle the information. Fortunately, I now have a great ophthalmologist who specializes in retina-related eye conditions. My ophthalmologist is frank and sensitive. He understands how important it is to preserve my residual vision.

—John

As the consultation begins, let your doctor know that you want all the information he can give you, no matter how disturbing. Tell the doctor that you understand that the knowledge may be upsetting to you now, but that you want to know all the facts. Explain that you feel you need this information so that you can begin to accept and deal with your vision loss. Then ask your questions.

Journal Note: A doctor who treated my knee injury was well-meaning but overprotective. Although I had tried every form of therapy with little benefit, he was reluctant to recommend surgery because he was worried about how I would function (even temporarily) with a double disability. Finally I broached the subject and, after assuring him that I would find a way to use crutches or a walker, the surgery was done. I truly believe that if I had not been aggressive and shown him that I could deal with the idea of a double disability, the surgery would have been postponed for a longer period of time. His attitude about blindness got in the way of his treatment.

—Vivian

But I Thought You Were My Doctor

Soon after your diagnosis or evaluation, your general physician or ophthalmologist may refer you to a low vision specialist or clinic.

This is not at all unusual and is done to provide you with additional evaluation, training, counseling, and low vision devices.

Most low vision services provide an assessment of your vision, a clinical examination, and prescription and training in the use of low vision aids or techniques. During the assessment information process, you may be interviewed by a social worker, educator, rehabilitation teacher, counselor, nurse, or other professional. This team of specialists may also provide training for devices or techniques that will enhance your vision.

The clinical examination is performed by an ophthalmologist or an optometrist. The exam determines and evaluates your visual acuity, visual field, functional visual abilities and limitations, visual behavior (including head and body positioning, squinting, and head tilting), attitudes toward optical aids, and motivation. Your low vision evaluation may take from one to three hours.

Your low vision specialists should be as open to your questions and concerns as your eye doctor is. You may want to arrange for a consultation with one or more of the people on your low vision team. You can use the same list of questions you took to your doctor or compile a separate list that covers your concerns about low vision instruction or services.

Information, Please

After your consultation, you may find that your doctor was able to give you a wealth of information about your vision condition, but was not as helpful about the resources and support services available to you. Even if your doctor was knowledgeable about local support programs, you may want to try to contact some additional organizations for further assistance and advice. (See the Appendix for a complete list.)

For general information, including materials on eye conditions, treatments, adaptive aids, publications, rehabilitation services, and resources for the blind, the following sampling of associations may be helpful. When you contact them, describe your *eye* condition and ask them to send you any information they have on your particular condition and sight loss. Most information is free or low cost.

American Council of the Blind
1010 Vermont Avenue, N.W., Suite 1100
Washington, DC 20005
(202) 393-3666

American Foundation for the Blind
15 West 16th Street
New York, NY 10011
(212) 620-2000 or (800) 232-5463

National Association for Parents of the Visually Impaired
P.O. Box 317
Watertown, MA 02272
(800) 562-6265 or (608) 362-4945

National Association for Visually Handicapped
22 West 21st Street
New York, NY 10010
(212) 889-3141

National Federation of the Blind
1800 Johnson Street
Baltimore, MD 21230
(410) 659-9314

National Society to Prevent Blindness
500 East Remington Road
Schaumburg, IL 60173
(312) 843-2020

Those of you who are legally blind may qualify for services provided by the following organizations. When contacting these agencies, ask for information about textbooks and other books on cassette, as well as books and magazines on flexible discs or records.

Choice Magazine Listening
85 Channel Drive
Port Washington, NY 11050
(516) 883-8280

Blindskills, Inc.
P.O. Box 5181
Salem, OR 97304
(503) 581-4224

Guild for the Blind
180 N. Michigan Avenue, Suite 1720
Chicago, IL 60601
(312) 236-8569

**National Library Service for the Blind
      and Physically Handicapped**
1291 Taylor Street, N.W.
Washington, DC 20542
(202) 287-5100 or (800) 424-9100

Recorded Periodicals Division
c/o Volunteer Services for the Blind
919 Walnut Street, Eighth Floor
Philadelphia, PA 19107
(215) 627-0600

Recording for the Blind
20 Roszel Road
Princeton, NJ 08540
(609) 452-0606

As you investigate available materials and adaptive aids, you will find that most are offered in braille or include braille markings. Although you may not know braille now, you may want to consider learning this language through formal rehabilitation or a correspondence course.

There are several types of braille. Grade one braille consists of the alphabet, numbers, and punctuation marks. Grade two braille consists of 190 contractions and is used for literary purposes. Grade three braille is another form of shorthand braille. There are special symbols for braille music, braille math and science notation, a braille code for computers, and braille for foreign languages. Braille reading and writing skills can offer many opportunities and are often required for some types of employment.

To learn to read and write in braille, correspondence courses are available through:

Hadley School for the Blind
700 Elm Street
Winnetka, IL 60093
(800) 323-4238 or (708) 446-8111

For books in braille, contact the National Library Service for the Blind and Physically Handicapped or:

National Braille Press
88 Stephen Street
Boston, MA 02115
(617) 266-6160

The National Braille Press and the American Brotherhood for the Blind also offer "twin vision" books. These books contain both braille and print that allows a blind person to read the braille aloud while a child follows along in print.

The American Brotherhood for the Blind
18440 Oxnard Street
Tarzana, CA 91356
(213) 343-2022

If your visual impairment is a result or complication of a disease, look in the phone book under the name of the specific disease for an organization to call (for example, the Diabetes Association, Multiple Sclerosis Society, Lupus Foundation, RP Foundation Fighting Blindness, and so on). Ask them to send you information about the disease, treatments, and local support groups.

While you are letting your fingers do the walking, look in the white and yellow pages for the phone number of your local Social Services. Also, check under the following headings: Service Groups, Human Resources, Blindness, Disabled, Department of Rehabilitation, Lions Clubs, and Fraternal Organizations for examples of support service organizations that have information to share.

If you have low or limited vision, you may be able to use a hand-held or page magnifier to look up the phone numbers. If this is not the case, call your local telephone information number (411) for assistance. (Information calls are free to legally blind persons in some states.)

Call your local library and ask about local organizations for the visually impaired. While you have them on the line, be sure to ask about their large print collection of books and magazines and books on tape. Also ask if they provide book taping services for the blind. Check with local colleges or universities to see if they have a Disabled Studies Program or a Disabled Students Organization that provides information and services to students and the general public.

State and Federal Assistance

You may be eligible for financial aid and other benefits as a result of your vision loss. This assistance may include Social Security benefits, state disability benefits, federal housing, special transportation, or reduced telephone rates.

Eligibility requirements vary from state to state. If you were working at the time you lost your sight, you should first contact your employer's personnel department for advice and information. You may then want to call the Social Security Department, Employment Development Department, and/or State Rehabilitation Department for Vocational Rehabilitation in your phone book. Ask them for information about financial aid, health insurance, and special services available to the visually impaired.

Depending on the state, the State Rehabilitation Department (in some states listed under the Commission for the Blind, Department of Services for the Blind, Division of Rehabilitation Services, Bureau of Services to the Blind, or some other agency) may provide nonvocational services as well. As a result of your particular condition or financial situation, you may automatically be eligible for government health insurance, aid, and assistance. Try not to let your sense of pride keep you from taking advantage of the funds and services available to you. You are entitled to them and using them may ease some of the stress you are experiencing.

Aids to Vision

Would a television screen that magnifies the picture sixty times be helpful to you? How about a talking clock that tells you the time and acts as an alarm or timer? Adaptive aids companies offer a wide range of devices designed to increase your independence and help you use your remaining vision in more effective ways. Activities that you thought were a thing of the past may be possible again with the use of an adaptive aid or device.

Adaptive aids may be beneficial whether you are totally blind, are legally blind, or have low vision. Although they may not improve your vision, adaptive aids can improve the quality of your life.

The following are a sampling from a myriad of available adaptive aid products. The market expands and improves daily. Some adaptive aids and devices can be ordered from adaptive aids catalogs, many of which are listed in the Appendix. (For more information on aids and technology, see Chapter 9.)

Magnifiers—standing, hand-held, around-the-neck, page magnifier, magnifying glass, sewing machine magnifier

Large Print—magazines, newspapers, and books are printed in large print. (Check your local library and the National Library Service for the Blind and Physically Handicapped for availability.) Other aids include devices with large print, such as telephone overlays, kitchen timers, and watches

Braille—a language made up of six dot "cells" that are read with the fingertips; magazines and books are printed in braille. (Check your local library and the National Library Service for the Blind and Physically Handicapped for availability.) Most aids for the blind or visually impaired are marked with braille

Indented and Raised Letters—letters of the alphabet indented or raised on paper for tracing and letter formation practice

Bold-line Paper—paper printed with dark, bold lines that are more easily seen than conventional types

Bold-tip Pens or Markers—pens that can be used to make large, prominent letters

Hi-Marks—a liquid paste used to make colored, fluorescent, hard, raised letters for writing notes or labeling items

Signature and Check Writing Guides—templates for signing signatures or checks

Letter and Envelope Writing Guides—templates with built-in lines for 8 1/2 x 11 inch paper and legal size envelopes

Raised Line or Large Print Checks—physical guides for ease in filling out checks

Label Makers—make large print, braille, and "talking" labels (recorded tape labels that are passed through a hand-held scanner that reads them aloud)

Raised Line Drawing Kits—produce raised lines that can be viewed or traced with the fingertips for making raised line notes, diagrams, or drawings

Talking Aids—watches, clocks, scales

Don't forget to consider the light bulb as an aid. For those with low vision, lighting may enhance their remaining vision. Experiment with placement, wattage, and types of light, such as incandescent or fluorescent light or high-intensity lamps. For instance, a 200 watt bulb and writing with a black felt-tip marker on bold-line paper may enable you to write letters independently. If brightness produces a distracting glare, it can be reduced by using buff or pastel paper.

> **Journal Notes:** Adaptive aids and devices can be useful to everyone—not just those with visual impairments. I ordered a pair of elbow-length oven mitts from an adaptive aids catalog because I like the protection they offer.
>
> —*Jill*

Taskmaster

How are you doing so far? Perhaps you have contacted a few associations and support groups, talked to your doctor, investigated financial aid, and ordered some adaptive aids, but you still do not feel able to function in your old routine. Perhaps then this is the time to make a list of your abilities. By examining your abilities, you will be able to define your needs.

For instance, when you realize that you can prepare food with a microwave or conventional oven just by marking the controls, you will learn that you need to have someone help you mark them. If you discover that you can learn to type through a correspondence course, you will realize that you need to find and contact a correspondence school. By listing tasks you can do, you will also uncover skills you would like to learn and this will lead you to new goals. By continually meeting current needs and identifying new ones, you will learn the skills you need to get back into a routine of daily living.

To start your list of abilities, divide it into four sections. In the first section, list all the tasks you can do without assistance (or after only a few sentences of instruction from a friend or this book.) You may have become so shaken by the vision loss that you do not even open a box of crackers for yourself anymore. Perhaps, in their enthusiasm to help, your relatives have taken over and do not allow you to do anything. List the things you can do and you may surprise yourself as well as your loved ones. Then—and this is the important part—do them!

In the next section of the abilities list, write the tasks you can do with adaptive aids. This may be difficult at first, but you will be able to expand this section of the list as you become more aware of the aids available to you. For now, use our examples as a starting point.

Next, list the tasks you can do with some assistance. These are things you feel comfortable with but just want a helping hand until you feel confident in your own ability. They may include reading your mail, taking a walk around the yard, shaving, or applying makeup.

In the final section, list all the tasks you can learn to do through formal rehabilitation. Include all the things you would like to be able to do but don't want to, or can't, learn from a friend or relative. These can be things you regularly did before your vision loss or new things that interest you now.

By now, you probably want to give your mind and body a break from thinking about and dealing with blindness, so be imaginative! If you have always secretly wanted to sky dive, ski, bowl, or play golf, don't give up that thought—include it on your list. (Yes, there are visually impaired sky divers, skiers, bowlers, and golfers!) By including interests and hobbies on the list, you will help to balance the effects of the trauma you may be experiencing relating to your vision loss. The following sample list will serve as an example.

Tasks I Can Do Without Help

wash my face (Chapter 7)

brush my teeth (Chapter 7)

comb my hair (Chapter 7)

take a shower or bath (Chapter 7)

eat using a normal table setting or serve myself from a buffet (Chapter 10)

make my bed (Chapter 7)

take my medication (Chapter 7)

get dressed (Chapter 7)

dust (Chapter 7)

vacuum (Chapter 7)

wash the dishes (Chapter 7)

clean the counter (Chapter 7)

sort clothes for washing (Chapter 7)

wash the clothes (Chapter 7)

identify coins (Chapter 8)

develop system for folding and organizing paper money (Chapter 8) prepare a basic meal - make sandwich, open packages and flip-top cans, pour cold liquids, make hot cereal and coffee (Chapter 7)

continue touch typing (Chapter 8)

dial the telephone from memory (Chapter 5)

ride a stationary bicycle

ride a tandem bicycle

work out in the gym

roller-skate and ice-skate

swim

dance

continue to play musical instruments

attend concerts, plays, sporting events

Tasks I Can Do with Adaptive Aids

keep track of time with braille (specially marked) watch, large print watch, or talking watch

write checks with large print or raised line checks (Chapter 8)

read books on tape, in large print, or with a page magnifier or optical aids (Chapter 8)

learn to touch-type through a taped correspondence course (Chapter 8)

touch-type (if you already know how) by marking the home keys (Chapter 8)

learn to read and write braille through a taped correspondence course (Chapter 2)

sign your signature with signature guide (Chapter 8)

address envelopes and write letters with writing guides and/or a typewriter (Chapter 8)

thread a needle with a needle threader or self-threading needle

use a sewing machine with a seam guide

heat food with marked stove, conventional oven, microwave, or one-cup beverage maker (Chapter 7)

pour hot liquids with a liquid level indicator (Chapter 7)

measure ingredients with marked utensils and measuring cups

dial the telephone using a telephone template or overlay (Chapter 5)

pay bills by electronic banking

play adaptive table games (Chapter 9)

play beep baseball

bowl using a bowling rail guide for the blind

play basketball by putting a bell on the hoop netting

travel independently with a long white cane

walk or run with a friend

Tasks I Can Do with Assistance

organize personal banking with a bank representative (Chapter 8)

identify and mark bills for payment (Chapter 8)

label clothing, food, and cassette tapes (Chapter 7)

mark settings on furnace temperature gauges, washing machine, microwave, stove (Chapter 7)

go grocery shopping

learn to turn off gas and water mains

use electric appliances—can opener, mixer, blender

Tasks I Can Do
with Formal Rehabilitation

all of the above

orient self and move about successfully in the home

apply cosmetics

shave

polish shoes

travel in the community using a long white cane, dog
   guide, and/or electronic or optical aids

take various forms of public transit

adapt job and choose vocational aids to accommodate
   vision loss

learn vocational skills

read using an Optacon or computer

peel, chop, grate food, cook and prepare complete
   meals

sew, knit, crochet, needlepoint

maintain yard and garden

wrap presents

learn how to use adaptive aids

touch-type

read and write braille

do home repairs and car maintenance

learn industrial arts

Now that you have made a list, you can begin to take the next steps. You may find that you need to contact an organization for visually impaired athletes or that you need to order a page magnifier. Use this list as a checkpoint for your progress. It will give you insight about what to focus on next and where you might go for instruction when you feel ready to accept it.

Keeping a Journal

Although you realize that it is important to express your emotions and feelings, you may be finding it difficult to do so. Maybe your timing has been off - when you were ready to talk, your friend was not available. Perhaps you felt that your son just was not able to deal with your complaints this week. Maybe in the past you worked off your feelings by going for a run or a bike ride, but you are not able to do that now.

Keeping a daily journal may be just what you need. It provides an outlet for your feelings and thoughts. It helps you keep track of positive and negative experiences, and it is there whenever you need it. You do not have to write about blindness. In fact, you do not even have to write. The important thing is to record a true reflection of your feelings.

Develop a means for keeping a journal. Perhaps your vision allows you to write with a thick-tip felt pen on bold-line paper. Later, with some study, you may be able to write your thoughts in braille. However, due to age or physical restrictions, such as a loss of sensitivity in your fingers, learning braille may not be an option for you. You may feel more comfortable talking and taping your thoughts on a cassette tape.

Use the journal to record how you react to situations, or develop it into a creative outlet and compose a poem or essay. A journal is also helpful as a problem-solving tool. By exploring the things you miss and wish you could do, you may discover other interests or alternatives.

For instance, you may mourn the fact that you can no longer ride a bike independently, but you may realize that you can ride with a partner on a tandem bike or alone on a stationary bike. You may regret that you never indulged your interest in wood-working and suddenly remember reading that your local rehabilitation department offers instruction in the industrial arts. Committing your thoughts to paper or tape can be just the catalyst you need to find a solution or realize the obvious.

Since your journal is a collection of private thoughts, you may want to write or tape when you are alone in order to maintain your privacy. You may need to impress on family members that this is a personal journal and that you want them to consider it private. You need not share your journal with anyone. To avoid having anyone accidentally read or listen to the journal, you may want to find a safe, permanent place to keep it.

To begin, set aside a regular time for making entries in your journal. You may want to make daily, weekly, or semiweekly entries. The number of weekly entries is not important but the regularity is. Make your journal a routine part of your schedule.

Set aside a time of day for thinking about what you will write in your journal. This could be when you take your shower each day or while riding home from work on the bus. Take this time to sort out ideas. Just let your mind drift.

Think about some guideposts to organizing your entry thoughts. You may want to separate your feelings into positive vs. negative, attitudes vs. reactions, concrete vs. abstract, dreams vs. reality, or hopes vs. fears. Include three things in each entry: the date, the time (you may be able to see a pattern in mood at different times of the day), and a goal.

Your goals can be immediate (something to be accomplished today or tomorrow), short-term (to be accomplished in a week to a month), or long-term (to be accomplished in a month to a year). By setting a daily, weekly, or monthly goal, you will focus on the future and guide yourself forward in the grieving process and toward becoming independent. It does not matter if the goals are unrealistic or seemingly insignificant. These goals are not etched in stone. You are really just brainstorming about what you would like to do—you are not committed to accomplishing specific goals.

> **Journal Note:** When I first became blind, my goal was to learn braille in six months. I accomplished my goal in eight months.
>
> —*Vivian*

"So if I'm not committed to doing them, why set these goals?" you ask. There will always be pressing goals you need to accomplish just to survive. But the journal goals will help you to focus beyond the necessities and toward more rewarding and enriching activities.

Sign off at the end of each entry. After all, these entries are a conversation between you and yourself so you need to end them as you would any conversation. Make your final thoughts as positive as you can. You may even be able to come up with a thought for the day. If you have had a particularly bad day, you could use the sign-off as a time to say, "Let's pack this day off in a suitcase and send it to the North Pole where it belongs!"

Periodically reread or listen to past journal entries. In doing this, you will see a revealing and comforting progression of growth. As you hear yourself say, "I just wish I could see what I saw a year ago," or "Today I made the bed without too many lumps," or "Tomorrow I'm going to learn to make a grilled cheese sandwich," you will be able to compare where you are today and realize just how far you have advanced.

Organizational Checklist

- Talk about your feelings with a trusted friend or relative.
- Prepare a list of questions about your eye condition.
- Make an appointment with your eye specialist to discuss your questions.

- Contact a counselor, therapist, or clergyman if necessary.

- Contact organizations for the visually impaired for information regarding vision loss.

- If your eye condition is caused by a disease, contact the appropriate service organization (Diabetes Society, etc.).

- Look in the telephone book under the headings: Social Services, Blindness, Service Groups for the Disabled, Handicaps, Disabled, etc. for support organizations and information.

- Call the local library and ask about large print books and books on tape.

- Contact the Social Services Department, State Rehabilitation Department, or employer about financial aid.

- Call adaptive aids companies (listed in the Appendix) to order catalogs.

- List your abilities and needs.

- Begin a daily or weekly journal.

4

Using Your Other Senses

Those of us born with five working senses tend to take four of them for granted. We often depend on the sense of sight to gather clues about the world around us to the neglect of our other senses.

You may need to start courting these neglected senses as you begin to lose your sight because, contrary to popular belief, you will not develop ESP as you lose your vision. This misconception has probably grown out of public ignorance about vision loss. Most people associate blindness with total darkness when over eighty-five percent of legally blind people actually have some usable vision. This is why sighted people tend to think something extrasensory is going on when someone walking with a dog guide remarks about the size of a passing pink Buick.

But it is not ESP that is working—it is just one of the usual five senses: vision, hearing, smell, touch, and taste. We included vision because, while visually impaired people must learn to use their other senses more effectively, they also learn to use their remaining vision.

Enjoy Your Other Senses

So take those senses out to lunch or to a show and pay attention to them as never before. Your sense of smell may tell you that the popcorn from the concession stand is particularly fresh today. Your sense of touch may tell you that the wooden arm rests have been worn smooth by thousands of happy theatergoers. Your sense of hearing may alert you to the number of people around you, the proportion of men to women, and the size of the room. Your residual vision may allow you to see the vivid colors of the costumes. Get into the habit of using all your senses as equal partners.

Your Home

These methods also apply closer to home. Assess your home using all your senses to be sure it is safe, so that you can enter feeling confident and secure.

When you enter your house, pause for a moment, look, listen, and sniff. Survey the room with a quick eyesweep. Does everything seem to be in the same spot as when you left? Is anything blocking your path? Is there a light left on?

Listen for sounds that should not be there, such as footsteps, running water, or street noises from an open window. Listen also for sounds that should be there, but are not. Is the clock still ticking? Is the refrigerator humming?

Sniff for gas or smoke. Does your dog have that unmistakable air about him when he rolls in the compost heap? Or can you pick up the scent of someone's aftershave or perfume?

Notice how the air around you feels. Has the heater shut off? Do you feel a draft from an open door? Does the air feel fresh or close and uncomfortable? Visually check or touch the top of the television or lamp. Does the TV feel warm? Is the lamp hot to the touch?

By practicing these methods each time you enter, you may soon find that you are becoming more and more comfortable using all of your senses effectively.

> **Journal Note:** As I lost my sight, I began to hone in on the voice of the person I was talking to. I listened to

his tone of voice, its intensity, inflection, personality, and volume. Now, I can even tell when someone is joking around because I use these clues coupled with the combination of words to fill me in.

—Vivian

People sometimes become so proficient at using their non-visual senses that they discount their remaining vision. They might say, "I hardly even look around me anymore. My vision changes so from day to day that I just don't count on it." This can be a mistake. Take advantage of the vision you have on any given day. If this means wearing lenses or using a magnifier or adaptive optical aid, by all means do so. Your remaining vision is valuable and will help you get the most complete information about your environment and surroundings.

Perhaps you are going to make yourself a healthful drink in the blender. Your remaining vision may allow you to spot the blender on the counter. You may be able to see the orange juice as you pour it in. Although you cannot read the word BLEND under the correct button, you may be able to recognize it because it is bigger than the rest or colored red.

When plugging in appliances in the kitchen, you may not be able to find the wall plug with the naked eye. But perhaps you can see it if you use a flashlight or if you change the switch plate to a color that contrasts with the kitchen wall.

Contrast As a Visual Aid

Be aware of contrast as a visual aid. As you set the table, you may notice that everything blends together when you use white plates on a light tablecloth. Experiment a bit and you may find that white plates against a dark green tablecloth help the plates stand out and be more visible. You may notice that white doorknobs on a dark door make it easier to find the knob. In a stairway, painting the walls adjacent to dark stairs a light color may prevent a fall.

Journal Note: Since I have limited vision and no depth perception, I rely heavily on color and contrast to orient me in and out of my home. When shopping, I tend to select brightly colored items. Since I experience difficulty in seeing red digital numbers on the black monitor, I purchased a calculator that has a green digital readout on a black monitor.

—*Diane*

When walking outdoors, visually check for landmarks or potential danger spots. Noticing the contrast of a green water hose in the middle of the sidewalk may prevent a trip or fall.

Journal Notes: For expediency purposes, I rode my bicycle to work rather than take public transit. I was able to bike to work in an hour and a half, round-trip. On public transit, it would take me an hour and a half one way. I wore safety gear and bright colors when traveling on my bike. I heavily relied on landmarks and colors for orienting myself in traffic. When I needed to check an actual street name, I would have to get very close to the street sign.

—*Louis*

Complementary colors also help. If you put a violet pull against yellow drapes, it may be easier to open and close them. (Those who are unable to see color should place tape on the pull.) To contrast other colors, remember that red complements green, and blue complements orange. Experiment with color, contrast, and lighting to enhance your residual vision.

Your Sense of Hearing

As you lose more sight, you may find that you are growing to depend on your hearing as a main source of information gathering. For this reason, you want to have the best hearing possible. It is a good idea to have your hearing checked regularly because you can have a hearing loss and be unaware of it. If you have a hearing loss that can be corrected with a hearing aid, don't allow something as silly as pride keep you from wearing one. Use it! A hearing aid can help keep you safe, and most hearing aids are virtually unnoticeable.

Be aware of the sounds in your home. Notice the normal creaking of the house at night. How does the fire sound when it dies down in the fireplace? What can you hear from the street when the screen door is open? Can you tell the difference between the bird scuttling across the roof and the cat stalking it?

How do the machines in your house sound? Every time you flush the toilet, take notice of the sound it makes. How loudly does the refrigerator hum? Does the ice maker make a crash in the middle of the night when it replenishes the tray? How does the smoke alarm sound in comparison to your alarm clock?

Listen for yard noises such as wind chimes, trees moving in the wind, sprinkler systems turning on, and neighborhood pets. Does Rover bark differently at the full moon than he does at a stranger? How does your neighbor's truck sound when he starts it up in the morning? What time is the garbage collected?

While walking in your neighborhood, listen for the difference in sound between trucks and buses. Be aware of someone approaching from behind. From the sound of the person's shoes on the pavement, could you tell the person's sex, age, or approximate weight? Listen for the direction and speed of traffic. Use your remaining vision to double-check the clues you gather with your hearing or vice versa.

Your Sense of Touch

Those who lose their sight gradually will probably use their sense of touch to confirm what they see or hear. When you are at the petting zoo and hear the bleat of a goat, you will most likely want to touch that critter at your side to see if it is indeed a goat. Touch will be even more important to you if you lose your sight suddenly. You will immediately use it to identify objects.

Touch will show you the shape, size, temperature, texture, and weight of an object. Your technique of touch can be sweeping—by trailing your hand along the wall to find your way down a hallway—or detailed — by holding cufflinks in your hand to distinguish the square links from the round pair. Your touch can help you focus your sight, too. For those with tunnel vision or peripheral vision, it may be easier to find an object with your hand and then bring it into the range of your visual field.

In everyday practical matters, your sense of touch can tell you that a washed plate is squeaky clean, a baby's diaper is wet, or your son has decided to give himself a Mohawk haircut.

If your sense of touch is dulled by neurologic problems, try to focus on what you *can* feel, not on what you *cannot* feel. When identifying an object, look for something that you can feel, such as a sharp ridge or a cold metal screw. Take special note of the size and weight of the object. If necessary, use your forearm or face to give you sensory clues about an object. You can use even the smallest amount of sensation to give you valuable information about your environment.

Your Sense of Smell

Your sense of smell helps you pick up a lot of visible and invisible clues. You can tell immediately if a room is clean by the smell, just as you can tell if a baby has spit up or dirtied his or her diaper. On the brighter side, your sense of smell can also tell you that the roses are blooming in your front yard or that someone is baking cinnamon rolls for breakfast.

> **Journal Note:** Although I use my residual vision and
> color for orienting myself to the environment, I use my

other senses to confirm what I see. Instead of risking catching my hair on fire in order to visually see if there's a flame under a burner I'm intending to use, I use my senses of smell and hearing to determine if it is safe.

—*Julia*

Use your sense of smell to warn you of danger. Be alert for the smell of smoke or gas in your house. A nice thing to remember is that when trying to smell something invisible, such as gas, you are on equal footing with a sighted person. In fact, you may become even more tuned in to such nonvisual information.

Journal Note: After a large earthquake, I thought I smelled gas in the garage where the furnace is housed. I got a neighbor to come and double-check for me. She smelled it, too, so we immediately left the house and called the gas company.

—*Vivian*

Smell also can give you information about people. With subtle sniffing you can probably determine if the person close to you is a smoker, if she is dressed up (wearing hair spray or perfume), or if he has just returned from participating in a sweaty game of basketball.

Smell and taste often work together to send you messages. Acting together, they can tell you that the batter is the right consistency but that you left out the vanilla. They will let you know that the milk is still fresh, the coffee is brewed, and the stuff you have squeezed onto your toothbrush is facial scrub, not toothpaste.

Try to think of the clues you gather with your senses as messages from five friends. Value and nurture them all, and they will serve you well.

Organizational Checklist

- Pay special attention to all your senses.
- After going out, get in the habit of checking the television and lamps for heat each time you return to your home.
- Make the most of your remaining vision by using higher light, color, contrast, and complementary colors.
- Become aware of the sounds in your home and neighborhood.

5

Getting Reacquainted
with Your Home

A man's or woman's home should be his or her castle. But about now you may be feeling like pulling up the drawbridge and locking yourself in the watchtower. You may feel intimidated in your own home—afraid of getting lost, knocking things over, or falling down and injuring yourself.

Even if you have partial sight, you may not be able to see the complete layout of a room and may fear bumping into furniture or destroying your own (or, worse yet, other's) valuables. These are all natural, reasonable fears. However, there are ways to reorient yourself to your home so that you will feel comfortable.

The extent of your vision loss and your attitude about it will greatly determine how quickly you can become reoriented to your home. Because of the wide ranges of vision loss, we approach this chapter from the standpoint that the reader is totally blind or has stable low vision.

The suggestions offered here may seem oversimplified. Our intent is not to insult your intelligence, but to present strategies for those of you at a most critical stage. For instance, you may have had a sudden onset of diabetic retinopathy, entered the hospital as a sighted person, and been discharged as a visually impaired person. These suggestions may not be too elementary for those of you who suddenly become visually impaired or are congenitally impaired but untrained. In any case, use these suggestions as guidelines and adapt them to your own visual needs.

Your Fears

To begin the process, you may want to examine your fears. What about getting lost? Well, suppose you do get lost in your house. After that awful first moment of disorientation, remind yourself that you are not "lost in the great woods never to be heard from again." You are, in fact, in your own home, safe and secure—if a little befuddled. You don't even risk the chance of getting rained on. You will eventually bump into something familiar and get your bearings.

> **Journal Note:** When I first bought my home, everything was so new to me. During the first week in my home, I spent a fair amount of time orienting myself to my surroundings.
>
> *—Vivian*

If you are worried about damaging delicate valuables in the room, you may want to consider moving them to a safer place for a while. After a time, you will feel confident enough to return them to their former locations.

If you are worried about falling or injuring yourself, you may be justified in your concern. You may have had a few collisions with the furniture and are wondering if it is deliberately sneaking into your path to trip you up.

Your problem is not sneaky furniture; it is disorientation. In order to feel comfortable and confident in your space, you have to feel a sense of boundaries and know where one item is in relation to others in a specific room. You can do this by reacquainting yourself with each room, using the sight you have left as well as your other senses.

Assess the Bedroom

At first, you may want a friend or relative present for moral support while you become reacquainted with your home. Ask someone you trust and feel comfortable with. If you feel absolutely paralyzed about moving through your home, pick one room where you will spend most of your time and orient yourself to it first.

Assuming this as worst case, let us suppose that you have chosen to orient yourself to your bedroom. One thing to remember is that you already have a lot of knowledge about this room. You know the furniture in it, its placement, and its approximate size. You know where the door is in relation to the bed. And, like most of us, you have probably walked to the bathroom countless times in the dark, so you have some sense of the distance to the bathroom.

Stand in the doorway of the room and talk with your friend about what you can see or remember about it. Perhaps you can see the bed or can determine where the window is by the light. Maybe you remember that the floor creaks just at the entrance to the hall. Point out the landmarks you can see, and indicate the general location of those you cannot.

Assess the room with the help of a friend. Look for potential hazards. Are there any pieces of furniture with sharp corners that are placed in the middle of the floor or along travel routes? Are there any wires, electrical cords, or rugs that you could trip on? Are there any low-hanging plants located along frequently traveled routes?

If possible, place the furniture along the walls or in places that accommodate your visual needs. For example, a light colored bedspread may provide a contrast to a dark headboard or furniture near the bed. A picture on the wall may provide a visual clue that lets you know you are approaching the TV.

It sometimes helps to move plants out of the way and to tape cords along the wall to keep them out of travel routes. The furniture rearrangement need not be permanent. Stay with the new arrangement until you feel comfortable moving about.

Now that the room is rearranged, choose a starting point from which to learn the room. Pick a place next to a wall. It could be the door leading to the hall, the bed, or the door leading to the bathroom. Always return to the same starting point when exploring a room.

From your starting point, stand next to the wall and lightly place the backs of your fingers on the wall in front of you. Sweep one foot in a semi-circle out in front of you. If nothing bumps your foot, take a step. As you move, trail your fingers along the wall in front of you and feel for changes in wall texture or breaks in the wall. Then repeat the process: sweep/step, sweep/step. You can use your free hand to sweep the air in front of you, first at head level, next at chest level, then at waist level as you sweep with your foot. This will alert you to obstacles above the floor level. You can use a yardstick in your free hand during the sweep/step method to increase the area you are exploring. This method of exploration will be replaced when you learn to travel with a long white cane.

As you travel, use your residual vision and your other senses to help you find your way. The shiny top on a bottle or the smell of cologne may alert you that you are only a few steps from your bureau. The slight sound of an echo in your voice could tell you that you are near the hallway door. The small rise in the carpet underfoot could be a clue that you are headed directly for the bathroom door.

When you reach a window, find the controls for the drapes, blinds, or shades. Practice opening and closing them. If you have two sets of drapes, identify one by placing tape or a contrasting color around the drawstring. Check to make sure that the drapes do not get caught on the furniture as they are opened and closed. If necessary, ask your friend to show you how to open, close, and lock the window.

You may want to memorize where everything is in the room. If you are partially sighted, this will enable you to fill in the gaps in your vision. Take several trips around the room using the sweep/step method until you feel comfortable moving about.

Once acquainted with the layout of the room, you may want to set up a work station in the room to keep together your most used items. A bedroom work station may consist of a large tray or cookie sheet where you keep your glasses, magnifier, daily medication, shoehorn, talking clock, cassette tapes, flashlight, radio, or anything else you need close at hand. Alternatively, you could keep these items in a drawer next to your bed.

Those of you who live alone or who lack a support system may still feel frightened to move around alone. If that is the case, guide ropes may provide a comforting means for getting around your home more securely. Cords or light ropes can be tacked to the walls with tape or small nails to help you find your way more quickly.

It is important to keep the guide ropes off the floor and to make breaks at doorways. Wrap masking tape near a doorway break to let you know that you are approaching a door, a step, or any other potential hazard. Do not feel discouraged if you have to resort to this method of travel. Look at the guide ropes as a temporary tool to help you bridge the gap to independent travel—like training wheels on a bicycle.

The Bathroom

It is unavoidable—you will need to find your way around the bathroom almost immediately. Fortunately, because it is small—and because we often use it in the dark—the bathroom may be the easiest room in the house to get accustomed to with little or no vision.

Make your starting point the entrance to the bathroom. Although you can probably count the number of steps to the toilet, start by following along the wall using the sweep/step method. If you have low vision, take a step-by-step tour, noting what you are able to see at each point. Notice the contrast of the bath mat to the floor, the towels to the wall, or the tub wall to the floor. If you are worried about slipping on the bath mat, you can tape it down or replace it with the nonskid type.

When you get to the bathtub or shower, take a few practice attempts getting in and out. If you have trouble getting into the tub, face the wall and brace yourself against it with your hands for support. Next, feel with your knee for the top of the tub. While holding onto the wall, step up, over, and into the bathtub.

Feel or visually check for the water faucets and locate their height from both standing and sitting positions. If there is a single faucet, it may have an arrow or indicator that points to HOT or COLD. You may want to mark the arrow with tape or glue, or scratch an indentation into it with a nail (more on marking items in Chapter 6).

To get out of the tub, just follow these directions in reverse. A metal handle or rail (available in hardware stores or adaptive aids catalogs) attached to the wall near the tub and a rubber mat or nonskid appliques inside the tub will reassure you and may help you avoid falls.

The biggest problem you will probably ever have in the bathroom is finding the toilet paper. The dispenser is often located in the most inconvenient and illogical place. So take time when exploring this room to practice finding the toilet paper while sitting on the toilet. Be sure to place extra rolls in an easily reachable place.

The medicine cabinet requires a little reorganization to make it accessible. Place the most frequently used items at eye level, moving the shelves if necessary to accommodate larger containers and visual needs. If you share the cabinet, perhaps family members would agree to let you have a shelf to yourself and to replace shared items to set locations.

You may want to make a work station for the bathroom. Place your cosmetics, soap, aftershave, mouthwash, washcloth, toothbrush—anything you need to find quickly and easily—in a separate drawer or in a container in the cupboard under the sink.

Consider changing the lighting in the bathroom to make use of any partial sight that you have. You may want to put in a stronger bulb or add a small fixture over the counter area. You may find that your particular vision is aided by dimming the bulb or replacing it with a low-level night light.

Kitchen Aids

Many people do not feel at home until they are in the kitchen. When you feel ready to cook up a relationship with this old friend, determine a starting point and begin. Pick a starting point at or near the entrance to the kitchen, and review what you can see or remember about the layout of the room. You may notice that the flooring changes from carpet or tile to linoleum at the entrance, or that you can tell you are facing the sink by the light you see shining through the kitchen window.

Next, use the sweep/step method to find your way around the room. Take note of how far it is from the sink to the refrigerator or from the oven to the table.

After you have the general lay of the land, visually note or trail your fingers along the kitchen counter to locate each appliance. When trailing, keep your fingers in contact with the counter and move slowly so you can safely feel the heat of the stove and hot appliances or the sharp edges of a knife left on the surface.

In an era when coffee makers look a lot like toasters to someone with limited vision, it is important to make a mental note of the color and shape of each appliance. You may be able to see that your toaster is beige and square as opposed to the coffee maker, which is black and rectangular. Determine where the appliances are in relation to each other and to the cupboards. By remembering that the toaster is just below the cupboard for glasses, or the coffee maker is just to the left of the sink, you will be able to find your way around the kitchen more quickly.

Until you feel comfortable locating kitchen items, a work station may help you find the things you need. Place a tray or cookie sheet on the counter, and put the things you use every day on it. Keep your favorite cup here, as well as coffee filters, a measuring spoon, salt and pepper, tea bags, instant soup packets, and anything that you need.

Your Kitchen Cupboards

If you have trouble seeing into the cupboards or are afraid of dropping glasses from the shelves, place the most frequently used dishes at eye level.

Drawers can be marked inside or out by tags marked with glue letters, cut-out cardboard letters, braille labels, talking labels, or large print. If you live with others, it is a good idea to keep one drawer to yourself for your most frequently used items or adaptive kitchen aids.

Your Refrigerator

The key to the refrigerator is organization. If you can remember to return each item to the same place every time you use it, you should have few problems.

If you are living with others, you may be able to agree to keep certain items in specific places in the refrigerator. For instance, it may be easier for you to find and identify certain things if they are kept on the door shelves. Encourage family members to return the items you use most often to the same spot every time.

If replacing these items seems too complicated for your free-spirited household, you could mark items you cannot identify by shape with rubber bands, braille labels, or large print or glue letters. (See Chapter 6.) For those who are partially sighted, storing food in brightly colored containers may do the trick. Do not forget to use your nose and taste buds to help you identify mystery foods.

The Rest of Your House

Once you feel at home in the bedroom, bathroom, and kitchen, you may want to become reacquainted with every part of your house. When you feel ready, go to your front door to begin the exploration process.

It is important to use the front door as a reference spot because it will most likely be your starting point whenever you enter your home. Practice getting to the front door from starting points in every room in the house. If you can do this, you will feel less frightened if you become lost in your house or need to exit quickly.

Learn to open, lock, and unlock your front door from both the inside and the outside. If necessary, ask a friend to verbally guide you through the process. A combination of your remaining vision and the clues you get from your fingertips will be the key to learning this skill.

Find the light switch next to the door using the door bolt or the doorknob as a reference point. You may find that the switch is just opposite the keyhole and up two finger-lengths. Practice finding the switch until you can do it easily.

When you are standing at your front door, take a moment to note what you can see and determine from all your senses. You may discover that you can feel a draft from the front door, that your voice carries a faint echo, that your feet tap loudly on the tile floor, or that you can see the bright red of the pillows on your sofa.

It is important to determine the safety hazards present in each room. In a living room or family room, furniture is often placed in the middle of travel routes. You may want to temporarily rearrange the furniture (especially those on casters) along the walls to help orient yourself and avoid bruising your shins.

Some people view bruised shins as a small price to pay for an attractive furniture arrangement, and there are other ways to ensure safety within a room. For instance, those beautiful throw rugs that you might trip over or slip on can be taped to the floor and used as landmarks to find your way to the TV. A low ottoman can be safely placed next to the wall to remind you of a step down to the living room.

To explore the perimeter of the room, follow along the wall using the sweep/step method. When you reach a window, determine whether the drapes are open or shut. Experiment with the drapes to see how they affect the lighting in the room and how this light meets your vision needs.

Continue to explore the living room until you have circled back to the front door. As you go, share with your friend or family member your observations about the shape of the room, the furniture placement, and the changes in wall and floor textures. Repeat the process several times until you feel confident that you are familiar with the location of things along the periphery.

To explore the center of the room, start near the wall, stretch out and use your arm-length to determine the distance between the wall and the first piece of furniture. Take note of distances as you move from piece to piece. It may surprise you to find that your coffee table is more than two arm-lengths to the sofa or that you have less than a hand-width between the side table and the armchair. Notice the configuration of furniture groupings. Do the sofa and chairs form an L-shape? Or is it more a semicircle or a square?

If you fear a close encounter of the painful kind with a piece of furniture, you may want to consider padding that table corner with a cushion or a toddler corner guard (available in grocery and hardware stores).

This is also a good time to learn how to operate the TV, stereo, radio, and other machines or appliances in the room. First, determine what you can see of the controls and what you remember about operating them. If you have any problems, ask your friend to help you fill in the gaps. If necessary, mark the controls with glue letters, braille labels, or large print letters.

> **Journal Note:** After my training at the Orientation Center for the Blind, an orientation and mobility instructor oriented me to my new home and adaptive aids were issued to me according to my needs.
>
> —*Rose*

The Telephone

One of the most comforting things about living in a technological age is knowing that help is only a push button away. Therefore, knowing how to dial the telephone is crucial. If you have some sight but cannot see the small print on the telephone, you may be able to see the large print on a telephone template (available through adaptive aids catalogs) or on the phones that now come equipped with large print dials and push buttons.

Regardless of the level of your vision loss, you can quickly and easily memorize the telephone dial. The push-button dial consists of three rows of numbers and a row with an asterisk, a zero, and a pound sign.

The first row:	1	2	3
The second row:	4	5	6
The third row:	7	8	9
The fourth row:	*	0	#

Find the first row of buttons with your index finger. Count off the buttons for 1, 2, and 3. Find the second row and count off the buttons for 4, 5, and 6. Find the third row and count off the buttons for 7, 8, and 9. Find the 0 button at the bottom of the dial, under the 8, between the asterisk and the pound sign. You may want to mark the middle button, number 5, with a glue dot for a quick reference point, or hold your thumb below the zero while you dial. Some phones have additional redial and mute buttons below the fourth row.

The numbers on a rotary dial phone are in a circle. Find the little metal, moon-shaped tab at the right of the circle. The first number up from the tab is 1. Count around the circle counter-clockwise (to the left) until you get to the last number, 0. This takes you back to the metal tab again. You may want to orient yourself to the dial by always finding the 6 first. It is directly across to the left of the metal tab. When dialing (assuming you are right-handed), always keep your thumb or the index finger of your free hand at the 6, then you can count up or down quickly to the next number needed.

With the phone unhooked or the disconnect button down, practice dialing phone numbers you know and 0 for operator. If your area has an emergency aid number such as 911, also practice dialing that.

Tape Recorders and Other Aids

You now know how to dial the phone and have even memorized the dial, but what if you need to call your doctor in a hurry and you have forgotten his or her number? Those with residual vision could keep a list of important numbers written in large print next to the phone. If you are unable to read large print, you can research the preprogramming options on newer telephones, write the numbers in braille, or tape important numbers on a cassette tape. You also can call the telephone company and ask if they will install emergency phone numbers on automatic dial.

Besides serving as a talking telephone book, a simple-to-operate, inexpensive tape recorder can be a very useful tool. It can help you make lists, keep a journal, remind you of medication instructions, and, of course, entertain you with music and books. It may be the best small investment you can make.

If necessary, ask a friend or family member to refresh your memory or guide you through the processes of recording, erasing, fast-forwarding, and rewinding. You may want to mark the control buttons with large print, braille, or glue letters. If you order a cassette playing unit from the Library of Congress (see the Appendix), raised markings will already be on the keys.

Record important telephone numbers (in order of importance) on a cassette tape. Rewind the tape and keep it in the tape player next to the telephone.

Safety Zone

Your home is your haven. You should feel comfortable and safe there, but with the loss of your sight, you may also feel a loss of security. Here are a few tips to help you feel more assured and safe.

- Keep emergency phone numbers near the telephone.
- Determine two exits from each room in the house. Practice exiting from each.
- Even if you do not use them to see, always leave a light or two on at night.
- Leave a radio or TV playing in some part of the house when you are alone. Leave it on a timer when you are away from the house.
- Light the front of your house at night. Trim any concealing shrubbery from the doorway and windows.
- Install appropriate locks to doors, windows, sliding glass doors, garage doors, and gates.
- Install smoke alarms and check them regularly.
- Memorize the sounds of your closest neighbors' cars or trucks.
- Learn how to turn off the toilets, water, electricity, and gas master controls.

Journal Note: When I first moved into my home, I called the crime prevention division of our city police department. An officer came to my house and evaluated it. She told me the kind of locks and lights I needed to install. I had arranged for a handyman to be there at the same time so he could hear directly from the officer

what he needed to do. The officer also gave me important information about the crime rate in my area

—Vivian

How Can You Help a Loved One with Vision Loss?

As a friend or relative of someone who is losing his or her sight, there is much you can do to help your loved one feel safe, secure, and confident at home. Assume an attitude of assistance, not dominance. Although it may be easier and quicker for you to do things for your friend, allow him to do things without assistance. Encourage independence and motivate him to try new tasks. Discuss fears, disappointments, and hopes.

Before you even begin the process of reorientation, discuss it at length with the visually impaired person. Find out what he or she wants to learn first and which rooms are most important. You can suggest tasks that are safety-oriented, such as dialing the phone and finding the front door. Together plan a schedule of meetings and tasks so he knows when he can count on your help.

Perhaps your friend is ready and eager to learn every room in the house. If so, start with the bedroom and bathroom, move to the kitchen, and continue throughout the house. Help him evaluate the safety of each room, find two exits from each room, and go through a trial run emergency exit.

Do not make decisions for the visually impaired person. If he wants to keep the elaborate furniture arrangement and learn to navigate around it, so be it! Applaud his sense of adventure and determination. Do not insist that all the furniture be moved against the walls just because it would make reorientation easier.

When he is ready to explore a room, allow him to place his hand slightly above your elbow while trailing the other hand along the wall. Slowly move forward. As he gains confidence, show him the sweep/step method and ask if he wants to explore on his own.

When he is ready, teach him how to use the telephone and help him tape emergency phone numbers on a cassette tape. Show him how to turn off the gas, electricity, toilets, and water. Help him trim the bushes in front of the house to make it safer. And do not forget the entertainment! Review with him the instructions to operate the TV, stereo, VCR, CD player, and radio.

If your loved one is reluctant to leave the bedroom, allow him that. But help him explore every inch of that room. As he gains confidence in the bedroom, he will soon want to branch out and become reacquainted with every room in the house. Ask if he would like you to set up guide ropes or landmarks as temporary aids to help him find his way around.

Encourage your loved one to do for himself as much as possible. You can even set up a one-cup beverage maker and a cooler in his bedroom so that he can fix himself simple meals (more about this in Chapter 7). This will help him begin to achieve independence and gain confidence.

Offer to help set up work stations in the kitchen, bathroom, bedroom, or den. Work with him to collect and organize the things he needs. Do not make his decisions for him. Ask which mug he wants on the kitchen work station—the large green one or the small blue one. Ask if he would rather put everything in one drawer or leave things as they are.

If he is hesitant to do things for himself, make it easy to be independent. Clean and cut fresh vegetables and put them in the refrigerator, or put instant soup next to the microwave so he can get himself a snack. Help label and hang coordinated clothing together in the closet so he can choose his own clothes each day. Go grocery shopping for him and assist him as he marks and puts away his new groceries.

Examine everyday tasks and consider how you could adapt the machine (marking with large print, cut-out cardboard, or glue letters) or the procedure so that he can do the task himself and further his independence in the home. Offer to teach him tasks, but do not insist.

If you live with someone who is visually impaired, try to

remember to replace items where you found them or to their assigned locations. If you find a door open, leave it open. If it is closed, reclose it. Close cabinet doors after use and replace furniture to their original positions. Keep travel routes clear and obstacle-free. Be aware of obstacles you may create at every level, from floor to head height.

> **Journal Note:** Other than keeping the household organized, remembering to push in chairs and close cupboards, I have not experienced emotional stress in watching my husband lose his vision.
>
> —*Linda*

> **Journal Note:** From the time my little girl was eighteen months until about three and one half, I felt like I ran into an obstacle course every minute. Now that my little girl is five, she is beginning to understand the importance of putting items back where they belong and picking up after herself.
>
> —*Diane*

When Time Is Short

You may be thinking, "I'd love to help out but I've only got a couple of lunch hours to offer." No problem. Here is a basic two-hour program that you can use to help get your loved one started on reorientation. During future lunch breaks, you can divide tasks and explore rooms according to his or her priorities.

Two-Hour Program

- Explore the bedroom.
- Teach your loved one how to use a tape recorder and the telephone. Practice dialing 0 and 911.

- Tape emergency phone numbers on a cassette tape or write them on a raised line drawing kit or in large print.
- Explore the path to the bathroom or put up a guide rope to it.
- Put snacks on a tray in the refrigerator.
- Set up a bathroom work station.

Organizational Checklist

- Obtain a cassette player and tapes. Mark the control buttons with glue or large print letters or braille labels.
- Record emergency phone numbers on a cassette. Place the recorded tape in a cassette player next to the telephone.
- Assess each room for safety hazards. Move furniture, tack down rugs, etc. as necessary.
- Identify two exits from each room. Practice leaving from them.
- Use a yardstick in the sweep/step method of traveling.
- Put up guide ropes for traveling in the home, if desired.
- Set up work stations in the bedroom, bathroom, and kitchen.
- Mark the bathroom faucet temperature indicator.
- Organize the refrigerator and the medicine cabinet.
- Place the most frequently used dishes at eye level in the cupboard.
- Label the kitchen drawers if necessary.
- Obtain a large print button telephone, a large print button template, a large print telephone dial template, or mark the number 5 button of the telephone dial with a glue dot.

- Install needed locks, lights, appliance timers, and smoke alarms.
- Provide cut fruits and vegetables and other healthful, easily prepared foods.

6

Changes in Family Roles

Since so much of our world depends on visual clues, vision loss will alter the way in which you function in the world. For example, you will learn to orient yourself using nonvisual clues. However, this takes time and you may need the help of others, especially at first. This dependence will often be centered on family members or friends.

> **Journal Note:** A loss of vision reminds me of an abrupt change of scenery in a play. You see one thing—then suddenly the curtain closes, opens again, and your world is completely different. It may take a while to reorient yourself to change.
>
> *—Vivian*

Your loved ones' reactions to you may take on some undesirable qualities. They may be patronizing: "Mom, you tied your shoelaces all by yourself!" or overprotective: "Don't worry about a thing, dear. I'm going to do all your cooking and cleaning. You don't have to lift a finger," or hopeless: "I guess now that you're blind the government will have to take care of you." Their responses may irritate you, but try not to be too hard on them. After all, they are part of a society whose first reaction is to protect a blind person rather than to further his or her independence.

You may be willing to let others do things for you at first, but eventually you will want to do more things for yourself. In some situations, you may need to prove yourself capable immediately. For instance, if you are a homemaker with young children, you may fear losing your children unless you can show that you can care for them. Or you may fear losing your position at work unless you can prove your fitness for the job. You will need to quickly assess your skills, abilities, and options.

To do this, make a list of: 1) tasks that you can still do, 2) tasks that you can do with limited support or help, 3) tasks that can be adapted, and 4) tasks that you will have to give up or trade for other comparable jobs.

Tasks that you can still do may include making breakfast for your children. Although they may be used to hot cereal, if you are not ready to use the stove or microwave, you can compromise and give them cold cereal and fruit.

If you feel uncomfortable bathing your children at first, do this task when someone else is at home and can help out if necessary. You may also ask for assistance in eliminating potential safety hazards in your house so that you know your children will be safe.

Are you worried that you will dress the little ones in plaids and stripes? Mark their clothing with braille clothing labels, embroidered stitches, large print, or a safety pin or straight pin, and you will still have the best-dressed kids in town. (See Chapter 7 for more on labeling.) With books on tape or large print books, you can still enjoy stories with your children.

> **Journal Note:** I am now 34 years old, married, and have three children. We took care of our children through foster care and were able to adopt them. My children are not embarrassed about having a blind mom. My children do seem to be overprotective of me, though. If anyone at school says anything negative about me, they're ready to beat up whoever said that. For instance, a child told one of my children, "Your mother isn't blind." And my child said, "Yes, she is."

The other child said, "How could she be, she can walk!"

—*Rachael*

Journal Note: I am totally blind. My husband is legally blind. We have two children who do not have any vision problems, a boy who is twelve and a girl who is ten years old. Other than asking our children to read correspondence or literature to us, our children lead "normal" lives.

—*Emily*

Unfortunately, you may not be able to drive your children to school, soccer games, or ballet lessons, so this is a task you may have to forfeit. Perhaps your spouse can take over this job and you, in return, can take over his job of making business phone calls or paying the bills. (Yes, you can! See Chapter 8.)

Journal Note: My wife is also legally blind. She has glaucoma. We have two boys, ages twelve and fourteen. Our children do not seem to mind having blind parents. They are very supportive in attitude and performing visually-related tasks like reading parts of the newspaper or labels at the grocery store. My wife's vision enables her to handle all our paper-related tasks. While my wife does the heavy housekeeping and keeps up the garden, I do the baking, wash the dishes and laundry, prepare our children's lunches, and do light housekeeping tasks. My wife and I both prepare the meals.

—*John*

In an office setting, you may find that you can still type and use the telephone, calculator, and other business machines by touch. You can ask an associate or a secretary to proofread your work for typos and misspellings, or you can use adaptive talking print scanners, computers, and other technology to assist you.

You may find that you can still read paperwork with the help of a magnifier and a bright light, and that you can read your own handwritten messages when you use a dark, thick-tipped felt pen. You may no longer be able to drive, but perhaps you can make prospective sales calls by telephone.

I Get By with a Little Help from My Friends

What do you do if you find that there are tasks that you can no longer perform independently? You probably will need to ask other family members or friends for assistance. Prioritize your needs and take care of the most pressing ones first.

Asking for help is difficult to do. Our society values giving, not receiving. Accept that you need help and learn to say "yes" and "thank you." You may even find that the other people in your life need to help. Think about those closest to you and try to determine who you would trust with each needed task. Keep each person's abilities and preferences in mind. Assess each one's schedule to determine how the task will fit into his or her routine. Most people will enjoy assisting you if you maintain a positive attitude and your requests are reasonable.

When you ask for assistance, be specific. Tell your neighbor that you need your daughter to be taken to school at 8:00 A.M., Monday through Friday, for the months of February and March. Or ask your mother-in-law to stay until the end of the month and tell her that during that time you would like her to work with you to reorganize the kitchen and adapt tasks so you can do the laundry, pay bills, and prepare simple meals independently. (See Chapters 5, 7, and 8.) If you can possibly arrange it, try to keep the time of the commitment to no longer than two months or so. People may feel more comfortable and willing to help if they know this is not a lifelong commitment.

Since your goal is to be independent, this giving of tasks to friends and relatives may rub you the wrong way. But it need not do so because you can reciprocate. If you are usually at home during the day, you can take over tasks that they dislike or do not have time to do, such as making phone calls or waiting for package deliveries or repairmen. You could pick up the mail and newspapers, water plants, feed the cat for vacationing neighbors, or spend time with their child who normally spends after-school hours alone.

> **Journal Note:** In terms of accomplishing tasks, my husband and I grocery shop together. He has a full-time job out of the home. I am responsible for taking the children to doctors and after-school activities. In addition to running my day-care center, I perform housekeeping tasks, prepare meals, and do paper-related projects. In exchange for my sister-in-law's child to be in my day-care, she assists me in performing paper-related activities.
>
> *—Rachael*

You may want to videotape favorite television programs or record music on cassettes so that you or others can listen to them in the car. Those of you with special skills will be able to do some sewing, carpentry, or typing with slight adaptation. Perhaps you can teach your support person how to knit, play chess, or cook your favorite exotic dish.

When you do your shopping, you may want to take along a support person's grocery list and do his shopping for him. While running errands, you can pick up another friend's laundry from the cleaner. Once a week, you can prepare a casserole or order some take-out food for a friend's family so she does not have to cook dinner that night. When you think about it, there really is a lot you can do in return.

As the two-month period comes to a close, ask another friend or relative to take a turn at task exchange. Thank your current support person and relieve him of his duties.

What do you do if your mother-in-law won't go home? Or your brother insists on doing your yard work even after you have told him you can now do it yourself? Or your neighbor insists on baby-sitting, but you do not want to leave your son in her care?

Admittedly, these are delicate situations, but do not be afraid to confront them. Make their role clear to your loved ones. After all, it is your life and you have the right to resume control if you feel aspects of your life are being taken over by others.

Tell your loved ones that although you appreciate all they have done, you can handle it now. Explain that you have a strict two-month limit that keeps everyone from feeling overburdened or obligated. Offer them a raincheck or assure them that you will ask them for assistance if you need it in the future.

For Relatives of People with Vision Loss

If you are a relative of someone with a vision loss, you may be concerned about several issues. You may worry about his safety. You may wonder if he has enough money to see him through, and if he does not, you may worry about the financial burden this will place on you. You may wonder how he will get his errands done. You may worry that he is not eating balanced meals.

You may be concerned about his emotional state. Perhaps your loved one is deeply depressed or is denying his blindness. You may feel that you can no longer relate to your loved one the way you used to. You may also feel guilty about the fact that you can see. You may be curious about how much vision he has, but feel uncomfortable discussing it. It is all so overwhelming—what do you do first?

Safety First

If your relative's safety is a concern, talk with him about it. Whatever concerns you have can be turned into positive action. Discuss what to do when a stranger comes to the door. Work together until he feels secure in locking and unlocking the doors and windows. Install smoke alarms and test them regularly. Conduct regular fire drills.

Check each room for safety hazards and work together to correct them. Write telephone numbers in large print or record them on a cassette tape and leave it in a tape player near the telephone. If long telephone cords are a hazard, invest in a cordless phone or additional phones in the rooms he uses the most. (More about safety in Chapter 5.) Develop a routine that he can go through at the end of each day to check for open drapes, unlocked doors or windows, switched-on lights, and oven or range burners that may still be on. A nightly routine check is an important habit to develop.

Making Ends Meet

Talking about money can be awkward. Perhaps your friend or relative will not even consider accepting money. You can still help. Discuss his needs. If better lighting would aid his remaining vision, perhaps you could pay for and install it. Or you can buy some plastic drinking glasses to alleviate his fear of doing the dishes.

On a more expensive note, a new microwave oven may be just what your loved one needs to safely prepare meals. You can also clip coupons for him to take to the grocery store or prepare a meal one day a week for him until he is ready to tackle this task.

You may give your loved one a lift to and from work until he can get there independently, so that he can resume working. You can do research on adaptive aids or training that would benefit him or find organizations that can support and advise him concerning his needs.

Medical Appointments

If you are worried about your loved one getting to medical appointments, offer to accompany him. Ask if he would like you to fill out the forms for him or take his prescriptions to the pharmacy and deliver them to him.

Perhaps your loved one refuses to go to doctor appointments or will not take medication. Take to someone more influential in his life to see if he or she can persuade him to cooperate. If this does not work, seek professional advice from a public health nurse or social services organization. Do not feel guilty if you have done all of the above and he still will not cooperate in his own health care. He has to want to help himself and will probably become more willing to do so in time.

If he has a fear of administering his own medicine or giving himself injections, offer to practice with him. You can help him to learn to measure the medicine in marked containers. You can also contact the Visiting Nurses Association or a public health nurse to teach you or your loved one how to measure medicine and give injections.

Emotional Roller Coaster

Your loved one or friend will go through a grieving process for his sight similar to that of a death. (See Chapter 2.) In time, he will pass through the stages of denial, anger, bargaining, depression, and acceptance. Through your contact with him, try to be aware of and sensitive to which stage he has reached. Your patience and solid emotional support will be extremely important to him, although you may question this at times if he seems to reject you.

If he is denying his blindness and refusing to wear his glasses say, "Gee, you seem a little down today. Where are your glasses? Do you think they would help?" If he replies, "Forget it, drop dead!" or something equally discouraging, offer to join him on a walk when he puts on the glasses.

In Your Neighborhood

When you go on a walk, choose a place that offers interest to someone with limited sight. Try to find places that include interesting or familiar sights and sounds, such as shopping malls, amusement parks, or nature trails.

On any outing, choose a spot with vivid scenery or movement. Even if your loved one cannot see everything, point out what he can see. He may be able to see the bright colors of the decorations in the mall, the breaking of the waves on the shore, the movement of a squirrel on a log, or the bright lights of sparklers against the night sky.

When you leave home, do not leave your loved one sitting in the car because his navigation skills are now limited. Use the sighted guide technique to help your friend maneuver safely and smoothly. Have your friend grasp the back of your arm slightly above the elbow. This places him to your side and one half-step behind you. This assures you of a clear view of any hazards. As you approach a curb or stairs, pause and say, "Curb down" or "Stairs up." As you step down or up, your travel partner will feel your arm moving down or up just prior to his need to make that same move.

As he gains experience in the sighted guide technique, your pause at steps will signal him to observe the direction of movement of your arm, and he will easily be able to tell when there is a step down or up without verbal instruction. When going through a narrow space, put the arm he is holding behind your back and he will follow behind. Of course, you could also say, "Skinny passage!" and he will get your meaning.

Back home, to help him combat denial, add aids that will help him make use of his remaining sight. Buy a brighter light if it will help him see his paperwork better. Get him a magnifier to help him read the newspaper, or make a regular date to read it to him. Check on available broadcast reading services for the visually impaired in your area or help him find out where he can learn to read braille.

You may find that your friend or relative seems angry all the time. He may lash out at you for what seem like trivial reasons. Remember that he is not angry with you, but with his situation. Try to get him to talk about it. Ask what is making him angry and what he misses most doing. Do not try to talk him out of his anger and do not tell him to count his remaining blessings. Quoting phrases such as "When life gives you lemons, make lemonade" does not really help. Loss of sight is a traumatic experience—he has every right to be angry.

Acknowledge your feelings, too. Admit that you are angry. Tell him, "I'm really angry that you are going blind. I feel guilty because I can see and you can't." It may surprise and comfort him to know the emotional impact his blindness has on you.

If he will not talk about his anger, provide an outlet for it. Engage in his favorite exercise with him, accompany him on a brisk walk or jog, and just let yourself be yelled at occasionally.

Try to put some fun back in his life. Read to him from a book by his favorite author. Take over a funny album or tape of a favorite comedian to enjoy together.

By now, he may be bargaining with God, the Fates, or his own personal Higher Order to retrieve his sight. He may say to you, "If only I had my sight back I would do volunteer work for blind agencies," or "If I could see again, I'd spend more of my free time with my children and grandchildren."

Remind him that these things are possible without sight, too. Say to him, "Let's do it anyway! You would make a great volunteer and with your business experience, you would be the perfect fund-raising consultant," or "You don't need to be sighted to be with your children and grandchildren. Let's find a game we can all play and I'll drive you over this weekend."

If your loved one is depressed, you may feel inadequate in whatever you do or say. If he needs time alone, respect this. Be patient and flexible. If you have planned to do something together and he cancels at the last minute, offer an alternate time.

Encourage him to try new things. If you think he would feel more independent preparing his own meals, mark the stove and microwave controls (see Chapter 7) and show him how to make basic dishes.

When he has a bad day and is discouraged, acknowledge his feelings and offer support if you can. Buy him a journal or an easy-to-operate tape recorder and encourage him to keep a daily record of his feelings and concerns. (See Chapter 2.) You may want to suggest professional counseling. Help him find someone with expertise in helping disabled people cope with emotional problems.

When your loved one begins to talk about his blindness and starts to resume some of his former activities, he will be showing signs of acceptance. You can show that you have also accepted his blindness by suggesting ways to help him be independent. If he wants to start cooking again, offer to copy a recipe in large print or to record it on a cassette.

Above all, do not be afraid to admit that you do not know what to do. Be direct. Tell your loved one that you do now know what to do and ask for some guidance. The words "Tell me what I can do to assist you" can work wonders to relieve stress for both of you.

Help Yourself

About this time, you may be finding the role of support person a heavy burden. This will be especially true if you are the only one of all your relatives living near the visually impaired person. You may feel resentful about your added responsibilities and angry that your loved one seems so ungrateful.

At this time you need your own support person. Find someone who will listen to your complaints with a nonjudgmental ear.

If you feel abused or manipulated by your visually impaired relative, tell him. Be honest and gently tell him when something is not working. If you have rearranged your schedule to take him to the park, only to have him cancel when you arrive, tell him that it would work better for you if he called and canceled ahead of time.

If he wants you to take him shopping when you have an evening tennis game scheduled, tell him that you cannot do it then but would be happy to get together at another time. It is important not to give up a time or event that you are emotionally tied to or you will almost certainly feel resentful.

But suppose that the only time available for shopping is during your regularly scheduled tennis game. You could arrange to do the shopping before or after the game so that both needs are met. Take your loved one to the game and let him enjoy what he can see and listen to the things he cannot. Chances are he will appreciate the change of environment and you will both enjoy this social time together.

If your friend or relative insists that you take over a task you do not like or feel comfortable doing, say so. Explain that you would rather take over his gardening chores and leave his laundry to someone else. Help him find someone who will do the task you have rejected, swap with another support person, or teach him how to do it himself.

If you feel that you are overloaded with tasks and need some help from other family members, it may be time to call a family meeting to discuss your needs and those of your visually impaired loved one. List the jobs that you need done and suggest members who can do them. Perhaps Uncle Joe can pick up Mom's prescriptions on his way home from work, or sister Sue can do Mom's grocery shopping when she does her own.

If you are the only relative living nearby, perhaps your relatives could be persuaded to pay for a professional assistant to take over some of these tasks. A small sum might finance the cost of hiring a college student who can take your mother shopping or help her do her errands.

If a regular sum of money is out of the question, maybe they could buy an item that would make your loved one's life more livable. For example, the purchase of a speech synthesizer for her personal computer may allow her to handle all her personal correspondence and finances independently. A new lamp or magnifier might enable her to read the newspaper independently. Brightly colored canisters to replace the clear ones she now has may enable her to find the coffee more quickly. Aids purchased from an adaptive aids catalog may enable her to resume cooking or help her resume playing a weekly bridge game.

If these things are not possible, perhaps visits can be arranged and scheduled to relieve you for specific periods of time. Perhaps cousin Ted can visit for two weeks in June and brother Sam can come for one week in July.

A Word About Words

Since communication is important at every level of transition, this may be a good time to say a word about words. You may find yourself worried about using certain words. You may have cringed when you asked your visually impaired friend, "Do you see what I mean?" "Do you get the picture?" or, as you hand her something, "Take a look at this."

Since the world is a visually oriented place, it would be counterproductive and insulting to deny it. Do not change your vocabulary for your friend. After all, "Did you listen to television last night?" does sound a bit strange, doesn't it? In fact, it may emphasize your friend's blindness.

Some words sound visual, but are not. For example, "Do you see what I mean?" really means "Do you understand what I mean?" and "I'll look into it" means you will gather this information and organize it in a meaningful way in order to make a decision. Conversely, people tend also to avoid the word *blind,* preferring euphemisms like *non-sighted* or *unsighted.* This is really an awkward avoidance tactic which, unfortunately, cannot restore vision.

> **Journal Note:** During my first phone conversation with Vivian I was overly conscious of her blindness and suddenly very aware of how many sight-related words are in our vocabulary. I winced as I blundered such

phrases as "Can you see what I mean" or "Look at it this way." She handled it with her usual sense of humor. When I suggested we meet downtown and stupidly asked, "But how will I know you?" she replied, "Don't worry. I'll be the only blind Black woman standing on that corner with a dog guide!"

—Jill

Ask your friend if he wants to be informed of potentially embarrassing situations. Does he want to know that he has a stain on his shirt? Does he want you to tell him that his socks do not match? When you do tell him, be direct and casual. If you are matter-of-fact and unembarrassed, chances are he will be, too.

Above all, keep your friend or relative in your life. Include him in outings and celebrations. Let him know that your love and concern for him have not faded with his eyesight.

7

Doing Your Morning Chores

Remember that old song, "Oh, How I Hate to Get Up in the Morning?" If this has been your theme song lately, give these suggestions a try. They may help you start your day on a brighter note.

When you first wake up in the morning, take a few moments to look at and listen to your environment. You may see the cat jump from the dresser to the floor, or notice that the sun is streaming through a crack between the drapes. You may hear the refrigerator motor running in the kitchen, the birds singing in your backyard, or your child stirring in the next room. Use this time to help center yourself in your environment and prepare for what you plan to do today.

Next, take note of your feelings. How do you feel today? You may feel like taking on the world. On the other hand, you may want to cry, scream, laugh, or pull the covers over your head and hide for the rest of the day. All of these feelings are legitimate and you may even find yourself swinging from one to another during the course of one day. This is natural and normal.

As you lie in bed, consider your feelings at that moment and acknowledge them. You do not have to take action on them, but if it feels better to scream or cry, go ahead. After all, it takes energy to hold these feelings in—energy that could be used to meet the day in a productive or enjoyable way.

Once you have focused on your feelings and surroundings, you may want to begin your morning routine in the bathroom (assuming that you have set landmarks to help you find your way).

The routine tasks presented here are basic. You can learn to do them with the help of a friend or relative. Later, under the guidance of a rehabilitation specialist, you will learn more tasks you can perform to take care of yourself and your home. The procedure we outline here is not the only way to do this. You can determine the approach that suits you best. The important thing is to adopt a routine and try to do your chores in the same order every day. Consider your morning tasks as the foundation for your day. Since these tasks are the most personal and familiar to you, completing them may make you feel productive and confident about tackling something new.

Your Teeth

Brushing your teeth is really a "feeling" rather than a "seeing" activity, but applying the toothpaste to the bristles may be a bit challenging. You can put the paste on your brush the same way you have always done if that works well for you. If it is difficult for you to find the bristles, hold the bristle part in your palm and lock the brush in place with your thumb across the handle. Then bring the tube over your palm and squeeze the toothpaste onto the bristles. This is a neat method since it is a lot easier to find and clean up excess toothpaste in your palm than on the counter or floor.

If you want to use a very easy, foolproof method, buy a tube of toothpaste that you alone will use (the pump types work well for this). Squeeze a shot into your mouth and brush. Simple, isn't it?

> **Journal Note:** Once, while visiting a blind friend, I needed to borrow her toothpaste. Unknown to me,

she had mistakenly reversed the toothpaste and another tube of medicine. As I brought the toothbrush to my mouth, something about the smell of the toothpaste made me hesitate. Good thing, too. It was Ben-Gay.

—Vivian

Your Face

Washing your face will seem less intimidating when you recall that you usually do this task with your eyes closed anyway. The only difference is that now you will use your hands to check the results instead of looking in the mirror.

Before washing, you may want to run your fingertips over your face to feel for oily or dry spots that may need extra attention or care during washing. Wash your face as usual, remembering to replace the soap and washcloth in their regular places when you finish. After washing, check with your fingertips for soap residue or areas you may have missed. Take this time to feel for any changes in your face, such as blemishes or cuts.

Your Hair

Depending on your hairstyle, combing, brushing, and parting your hair is something that may take practice to do well. If you feel uncertain about how you look, you may want to check your results with a friend. After parting your hair, you (both men and women) can temporarily put in a bobby pin, barrette, or another comb to keep one section of your hair in place while you comb the other side.

Your barber or stylist may agree to an appointment to teach you how to part and care for your particular hairstyle. If your present hairstyle is too much bother, changing to a simpler, more care-free style may prove less stressful.

Makeup

There are a variety of touch techniques you can use to know where, how, and how much makeup to apply. Although a sighted friend may be helpful, you may want to consult a professional makeup artist or rehabilitation instructor who specializes in teaching this skill.

Medications

If you take daily medication, you can distinguish one medication from another by touch or by using your residual vision. The size or shape of some containers should be enough of a clue to help you recognize them. Identical containers may hold pills that are recognizable by their unique shape, size, or texture.

To differentiate between similar containers with similar contents, you can mark the bottle with a piece of sandpaper or construction paper pasted to the back of the container. You can label it with braille or large print, or you can write the first letter of the medicine name in white glue or with Hi-Marks on the lid. When the glue or liquid dries, it will be a hard, raised-line letter you can read with your fingertips. Be certain, of course, that no one—including you—inadvertently switches the lids. If you prefer, you can mark a container by wrapping a rubber band, yarn, or string around it.

The important thing is not how you mark the medicine, but how well you remember the code you devised. Record a description of how you have marked your medicine bottles and the prescribed daily dosage on a cassette. This will give you something to refer to in case you forget.

Inexpensive pill organizers that indicate whether or not you have taken your daily medication are available in pharmacies and through adaptive device catalogs. Electronic reminders can be purchased for a little more money. The simplest solution is to invent your own method for remembering, such as putting the medication on the counter before you have taken it, and putting it on the shelf after you have taken it.

Your Bed

Making your bed is a great motivator for starting the day. (Why? Because you have to get out of it to do it!) You may find that making your bed is a snap if you remember to roll or fold the bedspread down to the foot of the bed when retiring each night. In the morning, you can simply smooth the sheets and blankets, then unroll or unfold the bedspread into place.

When you are ready to change the sheets, pull off the sheets, blankets, and pillowcases and put them aside. Next, take a moment to make a mental note of the height of your bed. Stand or kneel next to your bed and touch the floor, then measure in hand-lengths how high it is up to the mattress. It may be three hand-lengths or the distance from the floor to mid-calf. This information will help you accurately judge where to tuck in the sheets and blankets.

Now you are ready to put on the fitted bottom sheet. Locate the tag on the sheet. Place the corner with the tag on the bottom left corner of the mattress, tag-side down. Then put the other corners on the mattress.

Next, take the top sheet and find the wide finished edge that marks the top of the sheet. Take this top edge, line it up smoothly at the head of the mattress, and tuck it slightly over the edge. Put a pillow on top to help anchor the sheet in place while you pull it from side to side to get it even. When it is fairly even, tuck it in at the foot of the bed and along the sides of the bed. (Hospital corners? Be our guest, but frankly you needn't bother with them. We don't.) Follow the same procedure for the blankets.

You will probably find that putting a pillow in a pillowcase is the same task performed with or without sight. To put the pillowcase on the pillow, bring one short end of the pillow up to your neck. Nod your head down and hold the pillow in place with your chin. Your hands will be free to pull the pillowcase over the bottom end of the pillow. Once the case is tucked a few inches over the end, release the top of the pillow from its chin-hold, grab the hems of the pillowcase and shake the pillow the rest of the way into the case.

If you have neck problems, sit down and rest the pillow in your lap. After you tuck the pillowcase over the lower end of the pillow, grab the hems, stand up, and shake the pillowcase, letting gravity do the rest of the work for you.

Bedspreads and comforters differ in shape, but several clues can help you put them on correctly. Many bedspreads have rounded corners at the foot and square corners at the head. Most bedspreads and comforters have a tag. Locate it and memorize its location on the spread. Put a permanent marker such as a button or safety pin near the tag in case it gets torn off, or sew the tag down. Center the spread on the bed, checking from side to side, then from head to foot.

When you are finished, take a moment to measure how far off the floor the bedspread is on each side. Then next time you can place it four finger-widths (or whatever) up from the floor on each side and avoid so much moving about.

Dressing

Have you ever dressed in the dark and then noticed halfway through the day that your T-shirt was on backwards? Now that you have lost some vision, you may be worried about facing the world in mismatched socks or an inside-out skirt. The following tips will help you identify your clothes so that you can confidently put together an outfit.

First, go through your closet and see how many items you can already identify by touch or sight. You may recognize a shirt by its bold red and white stripes, a dress by its large, flat buttons, or a pair of pants by their generous pockets. Wear these clothes until you feel more comfortable identifying others.

Next, ask a friend to help you with the items you cannot recognize. Feel or visually check each item in your wardrobe as your friend verbally describes it. Those with usable residual vision can make note of visual clues, such as bold contrasts in color. If you lack usable vision, make note of special features such as buttons, belts, zippers, necklines, sleeves, and fabrics. Ask your friend to point out any unusual requirements or care that a garment needs. One may wrinkle easily and need frequent ironing; another may be sheer and need to be worn with special undergarments. Record these descriptions and requirements on a cassette tape or note them in large print or braille. These details will give you important additional information about your clothes, even if you decide to label them.

A simple way to label clothing is with a 3 x 5 inch index card. Use any white glue or Hi-Marks to write on the card. Make the capital letters BL for blue pants and BK for black pants. Letters cut out of felt or construction paper also work well for this. Punch a hole in the card and slip it over the hook of the hanger.

Hanging clothing on different types of hangers is another method. You can put the green blouse on a plastic hanger and the white blouse on a metal hanger to tell them apart. You may also want to hang matching pieces of an outfit together.

Just about now you may feel that you do not know if you are coming or going—but you do not want your clothes to reflect this fact. So, if you cannot tell the front or back of an item by touch, put a small safety pin or straight pin on the back. You can remove the pin when you wear the garment and replace it later.

To avoid mismatched socks, you can buy only one color. If you prefer a little variety in your life, you may want to tie a matching pair of socks together, or fasten them together with a safety pin, clothespin, or a plastic gadget made for this purpose. After wearing them, remember to pin them back together, then wash and dry them. (This trick also defeats dryers that like to "eat""socks.) Colored socks and underwear can be stored in a separate drawer from whites and sorted into two hampers—one for whites and one for colored clothing. This way you will avoid laundry mix-ups.

> **Journal Note:** One year I was a housemother for three children, ages 7 to 13. While breaking up an argument, I got distracted and put a red outfit into a white wash load. Although the argument died, the laundry dyed, too. Fortunately, the family was fond of the color pink.
>
> —*Vivian*

It may not be necessary to mark your shoes, since the texture, heel height, laces, straps, or detailing may provide you with enough information to identify them. Consider keeping shoes that are hard to identify in separate shoe boxes marked with glue or large print letters. The boxes will keep the shoes together in pairs and help avoid separation or loss.

> **Journal Note:** On the way to work one day a friend whispered to me that I was wearing two different shoes. They were the same color and the styling was only slightly different, causing me to put them into the wrong shoe boxes. I laughed it off as a new fashion statement, but decided to mark the inside of each of these shoes (and their mates) with braille labels to avoid a repeat experience.
>
> —*Vivian*

After you have marked your clothes, periodically review the cassette tape and update it when you buy something new. Go through your wardrobe once a month with someone who will check for wrinkles, spots, snags, or mislabeled items.

The suggestions outlined here are not the only ways to mark clothing. You can devise your own codes and procedures. Those who learn braille may replace the labels they are now using with braille ones.

Morning Coffee

Many of us cannot face the day without a cup of coffee or tea. If you fall into this category, you need not fear that you will have to do without. You can easily make coffee, tea, and a variety of foods using a one-cup, hot beverage maker. This reasonably priced, easy-to-use appliance is available through adaptive aids catalogs.

Put the beverage maker in a tray and plug it in near or on the breakfast table. The tray will catch any spills and keep water from dripping to the floor. Placing it on the table eliminates carrying a cup of hot liquid all the way from the counter to where you plan to sit.

To plug in the beverage maker or any appliance, visually or tactilely locate the outlet plate. With one hand, locate the edge of the outlet at the top. Hold the insulated part of the plug in the other hand and center the plug to the top of the outlet. Slide down the outlet until the prongs of the plug slip into the outlet holes.

It is helpful to keep everything you need to make your coffee or tea near the beverage maker. Your favorite mug, tea bags, sugar, powdered cream, soup packets, and a spoon can be stored on a separate tray or in a drawer next to it.

To use the beverage maker, fill a cup with cold water. Always work over the sink when you fill containers or pour liquids. To fill a cup with cold water, curl one knuckle of your finger inside the lip of the cup. Fill the cup until the water hits your finger.

As you may have guessed, this method does not work as well with hot water. When pouring hot liquids, place the cup in the sink. As you pour, listen for the water as it is going into the cup. You may be able to tell by the sound alone when the cup is full.

Another way to save your fingers is to use a liquid level indicator. This device has two short prongs that you hook over the lip of the cup. Pour the hot water into the cup until the indicator buzzes. This means that the water has reached the level of the two prongs. If you cannot hear the buzzer, put your finger on top of the prongs and you will feel its vibration. Liquid level indicators are inexpensive and available through adaptive aids catalogs.

Now that you have a cup of cold water, take it to the beverage maker. With your free hand, feel on the top of the maker for the lid to the water tank. Open the lid and leave your hand at the lip of the tank for a guide. Place your cup an inch or so above the lip of the tank and tip the water into the tank. Close the lid.

Next, slide the cup into the cup holder, then move your fingers directly up to the ON lever. Push the lever up and wait 90 seconds for the sound of a "click." (Those of you with some vision may also be able to see a light go on. If you cannot hear the "click," put your finger on the lever and you will feel it click into the OFF position.) Your water is now ready. Move the cup from the beverage maker to the tray, add a tea bag, instant coffee, instant soup, instant cereal, hot chocolate mix, instant noodles, or anything you like, and enjoy.

If you miss brewed coffee, you can easily use your coffee maker. Use your mug as a measuring device for the water and a scoop-type spoon you can level off with a finger for the coffee.

You can also use a whistling tea kettle or a microwave oven to heat water. However, some microwave ovens may be difficult to use, especially the type with flat, computerized panels. You can mark any type of panel with glue dots or Hi-Marks. Those who learn braille can replace the dots with a braille label or overlay. If your microwave is the type that uses pointers and buttons to set the dials, ask a friend to show you the timing intervals. You may find it easier to set the time with a separate kitchen timer or talking timer.

Timers

Most timers have a raised dot at the numbers 12, 3, 6, and 9. You can add a dot of glue at each number so that you will have a raised dot at each five-minute interval. Large print and braille timers, with dots at two-minute intervals, are available from adaptive aids catalogs, as are talking clock/calculators, which can be set for seconds, minutes, and hours.

Make a Clean Sweep

It's a dirty house, but somebody's got to clean it—and if that somebody is you, here are some tips for handling housecleaning chores.

Dusting

Put a pair of old socks on your hands to dust. You will be able to feel every crevice and curve on those carved table legs. Spray the wax onto one sock and dust, then polish with the dry sock. Work from side to side and top to bottom for even, smudge-free results. If you lack feeling in your fingers and are unsure of your results, just dust each area a couple of times. Draw a face on the socks and you will have an enjoyable way to get your children or grandchildren into the act.

Vacuuming

Since you already know how to use your vacuum cleaner, the key to vacuuming is to use a systematic approach. Furniture, walls, and windows may act as guides or reference points. To ensure that you have sufficiently covered an area, vacuum it vertically, then horizontally.

Washing Dishes

Wash your dishes just as you always have, but rely on your fingertips to tell you if they are completely clean. After rinsing, run your fingers over both sides of the plate to check for crumbs. Do this even if you have some vision. A bit of noodle, made invisible to the eye by an intricate pattern, will be easily "seen"with your fingertips. If you are uncomfortable with the idea of breaking a dish, you may want to air-dry them at first.

If you have a dishwasher, you may need some practice loading and unloading the dishes. Place a chair next to the dishwasher and sit down. You can then comfortably practice placing plastic or paper plates and cups in their proper slots. Put the knives and forks point-side down when loading them into the silverware basket so that you do not inadvertently poke yourself during unloading. After a few rehearsal sessions, you may even find yourself filling the dishwasher while talking on the phone.

Washing Your Clothes

This is an uncomplicated chore that you can do right from the start. Handwash your clothes as you always have; just add an extra scrubbing and an extra rinse to make sure that stains and soap are out, or let them sit and soak overnight.

If you have been living with ring-around-the-collar because you are afraid to use the washing machine, lay your fears to rest. Using the washing machine is fairly simple once you label the machine. Mark the most commonly used cycles on the dials with large print, glue, braille or Hi-Mark letters (PP for permanent press, H for hot, and so on). The letters will show you where to set the pointer for the desired temperature, time setting, and water level.

If your machine does not have a pointer as a setting device, you can create one. Put a glue or Hi-Mark dot on the setting device and a dot at the beginning of each cycle on the dial. To set the cycle, just match the two dots.

Many washing machines have a built-in measuring cup. If yours does not, keep a nonbreakable measuring cup or spoon next to the laundry soap. You may also want to keep your soap measurements recorded on a cassette tape.

You can label the dryer's cycles, too. Put glue, Hi-Mark, braille, or cut-out cardboard or paper letters on the fabric and time selector dials. If necessary, put dots on the setting device and at the beginning point of each cycle.

Feel each item when you load the clothes into either machine. The texture and type of garment will supply clues about the fabric. This, along with the separate clothes hampers for colored and white clothes, should help you avoid any mishaps.

Journal Note: Most tasks only require adaptive techniques and organization to accomplish. While in student teacher training, I supported myself by cleaning a house for a professor and his family. I was responsible for general cleaning, keeping up hardwood floors, preparing vegetables and fruit for the week, doing laundry and ironing. During the interview for the job, the couple was concerned about how I would iron. I explained to them that, other than following the cord up to locate the handle, my method of ironing is no different from a sighted person's. I further indicated that rather than ironing by sight, I iron by touch.

—Vivian

Countertops

When you are ready to clean the countertop, feel it with your fingers first to compare it with the results when you are finished. Put any canisters or other counter items on a cookie sheet or systematically move them aside, then clean from back to front, or from side to side. Check the cleaned counter with your fingertips, replacing each item as you finish cleaning that section. This will help you keep track of where you have cleaned.

Spills

Into each life a little rain must fall, along with a little milk, a little coffee, and a lot of Cheerios. If you find yourself facing a counter spill, use your fingertips or residual vision to find its boundaries. Wipe the area with a sponge or towel, then visually check or feel the cleaned counter for spots you may have missed. Feel or look at the wall below the counter and the floor, then wipe any spills you find.

If the spill contains broken glass, move cautiously and assume that there may be glass on the floor. Get a wastebasket, some towels, and a bowl.

Carefully remove any counter items and put them in the sink or into the bowl. Place the towels over the spill. Hold the wastebasket at the edge of the counter and move each towel toward the basket, sliding the spill and the glass into it. Gently shake each towel into the basket to remove the glass. Put the towels into a plastic or paper bag until either you or a friend or relative can thoroughly check them.

Gently wipe the counter again with a sponge or towel and listen for the scraping sound of glass fragments on the surface. Wipe the counter items and replace them.

When you spill something on the floor, stop immediately and look and listen for where the liquid or glass has gone. Carefully feel for the boundaries of the spill. Get some towels and put them over the spill. If it is only liquid, wipe it up.

If the spill contains broken glass, get a wastebasket and set it on its side near the spill. Slide the towels to the edge of the basket, and ease the glass and liquid in. Repeat the process several times, checking with your fingertips between wipings. Shake the towels into the basket and put them in a plastic bag so you or a friend or relative can do a visual or tactile check later.

You may feel uncomfortable, afraid, or just too tired some days to deal with a major spill. If so, cover the spill with towels and avoid the area until someone can assist you.

Take a Bow

If you have completed any of these tasks today, even if it was simply rolling out of bed, give yourself a pat on the back. You have made a start. As you learn to do one chore, you will gain confidence and that will lead to doing more. You do not need to add a new accomplishment each day. In fact, you may have days when you can do very little and will feel as though you are regressing.

When you have had a good day, share it with someone. Call a friend or relative and crow a little. But also, when you've spilled the coffee, lost your shoe, or squirted yourself in the eye with toothpaste (and it's only 10:00 A.M.), share that with someone, too. Don't be afraid to complain. Do so, then get on with your conversation and your day.

If you are a relative or friend of a visually impaired person, you can offer encouragement and humor. When your friend makes coffee for the first time, you might present her with a brand new, gift-wrapped can of her favorite coffee. Children and grandchildren can make paper medals or ribbons to commemorate each achievement and show their pride. Look for opportunities for small celebrations. Life is full of them.

Allow your loved one to gripe a bit on discouraging days. He will probably feel better when you agree that "It really is the pits trying to find the doorway in the dark." You might even consider trying some of these tasks blindfolded. It will give you a taste of what your friend or relative is experiencing, and will also increase your understanding.

After acknowledging your loved one's complaints, try to turn the conversation to a more positive tone. Remind him of his accomplishments, recognize his perseverance, and suggest that toothpaste may be a great new makeup remover! A little humor never hurts.

You can also help your visually disabled friend make some changes in his or her home that can make daily tasks easier to do. These changes can be made all at once or one at a time. You might help rearrange a kitchen drawer this week, and your son might help organize the bathroom next week. However it is done, use this time to socialize with and support your loved one.

Organizational Checklist

Kitchen

- Set aside a drawer, counter space, or a tray for food preparation items, such as a cup, spoon, tea bags, or liquid level indicator.

- Place the most frequently used electrical appliances near accessible outlets.

- Place similar items together in a cupboard near where they will be used—all spices on one shelf near the stove, all cooking utensils on another, and so on.

- If space is a problem, divide the shelves with tall food boxes. You can put cereals on one side, canned goods on the other.

- Store all microwave cookery near the microwave oven.

- Place all storage bowls for leftovers near the refrigerator.

- Place a plastic mat in the sink to cushion dropped plates.

- Organize the drawers by use. Place all stove utensils next to the stove, etc.

- Arrange things used during meals on the dining table, including napkin rack, salt and pepper, etc.

- Mark canned goods and food containers with large print or braille, or glue letters on 3 x 5 inch cards for identification. Attach the cards with a rubber band or tape.

- Those with some vision can enlarge the print on food containers with a bold-tip marking pen. Use capital letters.

- Those who learn braille can label food containers with 3 x 5 inch cards secured to the containers with a rubber band.

- Refer to *Suggestions for the Blind Cook* by Ruth Schroeder (see the Bibliography) for cooking tips.

Bathroom

- Set aside a drawer or two shelves in the medicine cabinet for toothbrush, toothpaste, shampoo, etc.

- Replace a glass cup with a plastic cup or a paper cup dispenser.

- Place a rubber mat in the bathtub or shower.

- Keep toilet paper rolls within easy reach of the toilet.

- Create a carry-all container of toiletries (deodorant, talc, shower cap, etc.) and keep it in the bathroom or bedroom.

Bedroom

- Organize the dresser drawers, separating colored clothing from whites.

- Set aside a drawer or tray for cosmetics or hair care items.

- Place two laundry hampers (or baskets, boxes, etc.) in the room or in the closet. Use one for colored clothing, one for whites.

- Place a clock (braille, large print, talking, or one that you can read with your fingertips) on the nightstand.

- Place the telephone within reach of your bed.

- Place a cassette player with phone numbers next to the phone.

- Place a flashlight and a battery-operated radio within reach of your bed in case of power outages or shortages.

Office or Family Room

- Set up a small table or work space for sighted persons who will help with paperwork. Provide envelopes, stamps, pens, etc.

- Organize a backpack or carry-all for a tape recorder, cassettes, talking calculator, (a cane, when you are ready to use one) and other items that travel from room to room or away from home.

8

Handling Your Paperwork

Undeterred by rain or sleet or dark of night, your mail keeps coming. Even if you can read large print or some standard print, you may soon feel awash in a sea of mail, praying for a federal holiday to stop the flow.

Since we value our privacy so highly—after all, in order to protect your privacy, the government has ruled that it is a federal offense to open anyone else's mail—loss of control of your private and business correspondence due to vision loss can be a main source of depression.

But never fear—you do not have to turn your mail, money affairs, business correspondence, or personal letters over to someone else. You can take steps to organize your mail and business papers to give you maximum control and privacy for your personal needs.

Sorting Your Mail

Begin by sorting your mail when it arrives each day. If you have some vision, you may be able to use a magnifier to identify each piece. If not, feel or visually check each piece of mail, sorting the envelopes into one pile and everything else into another. Much of the pile that does not contain envelopes will consist of low priority mail—fliers and ads that do not require your immediate attention.

If there is a bill you want to distinguish immediately from all the others, call the biller and ask to have something done to the bill that will set it apart from the others. Perhaps sending it in an over-long envelope with a staple or fold in it or with a large visual sign like a check mark or X in one corner would do it—anything that will enable you to identify it by touch or sight.

> **Journal Note:** I needed to identify a bill from my doctor right away, so I called and asked the receptionist to put a small piece of scotch tape on the bottom right corner of the envelope. When the bill arrived, I was able to recognize it immediately.
>
> —*Vivian*

Wrap each pile of mail with a rubber band or put each group in separate envelopes. Mark the date on the pile or envelope with large print, glue letters, on a 3 x 5 inch card, cut-out cardboard letters, braille, or talking labels, and file or shelve it in order of delivery date. This way, you can attack the mail in priority order when you have assistance.

If you start to feel overwhelmed, get the phone numbers (call 411 for telephone assistance if necessary) of your billing companies and record them on a cassette. Then call to see if they will temporarily hold your mail for you. Ask if you can do your business over the telephone.

Although you have now started to organize your mail, you still may be wondering how many bills are in those envelopes and when are they due. Even if you are currently up to date financially, you may feel anxious about not being able to see your bills and pay them by yourself. This is the time to think about someone you can trust to help you.

> **Journal Note:** I handle my mail on a week-by-week basis. I either have my adult children or a trusted friend read my mail to me. Privacy has been a big issue for me.
>
> —*Janice*

Trusty Assistant

Relatives often will offer or be willing to assist you with your mail and bills. If you feel comfortable with this, accept their offers of assistance or ask a particular loved one to assist you. If you do not want your relatives to know your private business, you will need to ask a trusted friend or consider hiring someone to assist you with this task. No matter who you choose, you will probably feel some resentment about your loss of privacy.

For Friends and Relatives

If you are a friend or relative assisting with the mail or bills, you can encourage your loved one to take an interest in financial matters. Read all mail and business correspondence aloud and do not keep secrets from him—no matter how distressing. Do not make any decisions or take any action without conferring with your loved one.

Take each session slowly and easily. If you cannot do all the bills in one session, schedule two or more less lengthy (and less stressful) sessions. Your encouragement in this area will do much to make your loved one feel independent and in control of his or her life.

Down to Business

Even if you decide to ask a friend or relative for assistance, there are many aspects of your financial affairs that you can direct without their involvement. Do not automatically assume that someone else needs to do everything for you. Explore other possibilities.

In some cases, you may be able to pay your bills at the place of business. For instance, you may be able to pay your monthly pharmacy bill while in the drugstore picking up a prescription. Your monthly gas and electricity bills may be paid similarly. When paying by check, ask the clerk to help you fill in the amount if you need assistance and show you where to sign. Whenever possible, fill out your check in advance.

> **Journal Note:** Asking someone to help you fill in a check will feel strange the first few times. You will feel very vulnerable. But I've had people do this for me hundreds of times and have never once been cheated. In fact, people bend over backward to prove to you that they are honest. In the grocery store once, the clerk filled out the check then called someone over to verify that he had written it as asked. "I trust you, I trust you," I said. I think he felt even more vulnerable than I did.
>
> —*Vivian*

Those of you who touch-type may want to mark the two home reference keys, F and J, with glue or felt dots. This may allow you to type the amount of the check and you can later have your assistant double-check it for typos or misspellings. Your usable residual vision may allow you to complete your present checks with the help of a magnifier and bold-tip felt pen.

Many banks offer raised line or large print checks, and adaptive aids catalogs list standard check templates and some that can be made to order. Or you can cut windows into a piece of cardboard to create a homemade template. These aids may allow you to fill out your checks independently. Later, you may be able to handle all of your financial affairs independently with the use of electronic aids such as an Optacon, closed circuit TV, computer braille, electronic reading machines with speech synthesizers, or other devices. (See Chapter 9.)

> **Journal Note:** I am able to perform most paper-related tasks independently. My checks have dark, wide lines and are in large print. Instead of risking placing the address portion of the bill upside down in the window of the envelope, I always check with a sighted

friend to confirm that my bills are appropriately addressed.

—Rose

In the meantime, if you want to stay in charge, do not let your assistant take the checks home and pay them. Insist that you be present so that you are aware of each check you sign. Although their motives may be well-meaning, family members can often take control away from you in this way. This is avoidable if you set limits and guidelines. This is your own personal business, and you can still be in charge.

Set up a place in your home for working with an assistant and for organizing paper projects. You do not need a formal office. You can use a section of the kitchen table, a card table set up in the bedroom, or a set of shoebox files on an organizing tray. You will need a place for both you and your assistant. There is less chance and less temptation for your assistant to get into your personal papers if he has a separate work space. Do not let your assistant take over your desk. Set aside a smaller table next to your desk, or clear half of your desk for his or her use.

Gather the tools the assistant will need: pens, pencils, erasers, paper clips, a writing light, rubber bands, address stickers, stapler, signature guide or cardboard or "Post-it" note to serve as a signature guide, address book, paper, stapler, envelopes, stamps, and so on.

At your work space, you may need a signature guide, cassette tapes, recorder, card file, typewriter, bold-line paper, label maker, bold-tip felt pen, raised line paper, raised line or large print checks, check templates, letter writing guide, magnifier, talking calculator, and so on.

Your Signature

You may have noticed that a signature stamp was not included in either list. Although this may appear to be a wonderful aid, the long-term consequences of its use can be serious. We urge you to think long and hard before adopting this method. Signature stamps are often unnecessary. You may assume that you cannot write your name without your sight, but remember that you write your signature fairly automatically. The problem is not so much *how* to write your signature, but where and what size to write it. You can efficiently sign your name with the help of a signature guide or a piece of cardboard laid under the signature line.

> **Journal Note:** I find that a stack of "Post-it" notes works great as a substitute for a signature guide, since it sticks in place and doesn't move.
>
> *—Vivian*

Do not be concerned if your signature is not perfect. Anyone who has tried to read a prescription knows that it is the form and style that counts, not the legibility. If you still have doubts, you may want to practice tracing on raised line letters or in indented letters. Both come on sheets available through adaptive aids catalogs (listed in the Appendix). You can also practice on a small chalkboard while watching TV or during other leisure moments. If you need a quick reminder about a certain letter, have a friend move your hand in the formation of the letter several times until it comes back to you.

Ground Rules
When Working with an Assistant

The first time you sit down with your assistant, you may want to set some ground rules to avoid any misunderstandings or hurt feelings. If you want to retain control of your finances, say so. Explain that you are grateful for this support but that you want to stay in complete knowledge and control of your affairs.

Describe what you want your assistant to do: open mail, identify bills, read business correspondence to you, write checks or help you to do so, assist you in signing checks and documents, update and reconcile your checkbook, and so on.

Have your assistant help you set up a record-keeping system during the first month of bill-paying sessions. Write in large print or tape on a cassette the date each bill arrives. This way you will know when to expect it each month. Your assistant can start with the oldest bills from your daily mail bundles and begin to help you pay them. You and your assistant can write the check amounts and you can sign the checks.

> **Journal Note:** Although I can write checks independently with a typewriter, it's not a high priority for me to do them myself. I have an assistant write them while I'm in the room doing other paperwork. I can follow the assistant's progress by listening to my talking calculator as she works.
>
> *—Vivian*

To write your signature in the appropriate place, ask your assistant to place a piece of cardboard, a signature template, or a stack of "Post-it" notes under the line where you will sign. To show you how long the signature line is, ask your assistant to place his finger or your finger at the end of the line. Then, sign away.

As each bill is paid, put it back in the original envelope and mark the name and date of the bill on the envelope with large print, glue letters, or braille on a 3 x 5 inch card. By handling these envelopes each month, you will soon be able to identify certain bills by the envelope size, window location, color, or type of paper.

Put the marked envelopes into a large manila or closable file folder (to avoid problems if dropped) marked **PAID BILLS**. These can also be filed under additional categories, such as **Rent** or **Mortgage**, **Gas**, **Electric**, **Water**, **Visa**, **Mastercard**, and so on. Those bills you do not get to can be filed in an envelope or folder marked **UNPAID BILLS**, and you can pay them at the next session. File these in a file cabinet, shelf, or shoebox—anything that works for you.

You might mark additional folders or envelopes as follows: **PERSONAL CORRESPONDENCE, BUSINESS CORRE-SPONDENCE, CANCELED CHECKS 1/92 to 1/93, INSURANCE, MEDICAL RECORDS, WARRANTIES**, and so on. If you already have a filing system, mark the envelopes in large print, braille, glue letters, talking labels, etc., to make them more accessible. As an alternative, mark paid bills with a rubber band and unpaid bills with a paper clip and then file them in a shoe box.

> **Journal Note:** I handle paperwork in a variety of ways. I use a closed circuit television to scan my mail. I hire someone to read specific mail items to me. I always keep my bills in one place. I use the closed circuit television, along with a check writing guide, for paying bills. I label my bills in large print and/or in braille. Since my vision changes from day to day, I usually rely on braille for documenting important matters.
>
> —*Julia*

Having a Stranger in Your House

If you must hire a stranger to assist you with paper-related projects, you can take steps so that you will feel safe and confident about your assistant. When someone contacts you from an agency, get his or her name, address, and phone number. Call information (411) or get the agency phone number from the telephone book and call to verify this person's employment and to get a general physical description of the person.

When the appointment is made, ask a neighbor to watch for the arrival of a person of that description at the appropriate time. Ask your neighbor or a friend to call or "drop by" if the person who arrives is different from the description. Hide your purse or valuables. Leave one exit door unlocked. Ask for the person's name and agency name before opening the door. Wait until you are at the door before asking for identification—you may be distracted from listening while trying to find your way to the door.

Start to gain trust in your assistant slowly. At first, give him or her things to do that are not personal. During the first meeting, ask your assistant to fill out an employee information form. Some of the questions on the form may include name, address, phone number, Social Security number, driver's license number, car license number, educational status, and previous work experience or references.

> **Journal Note:** The first time I meet with a new assistant, I arrange for a friend to drop by during the first day of work. My friend then can provide some nonverbal feedback, as well as verify information on the form.
> —*Vivian*

Handling Money

Mail is not the only paper that needs your attention. There is one type of paper that you handle almost everyday - money.

Most people develop their own system for identifying and separating their money. Some prefer to keep groups of the same denomination together with a paper clip or rolled up in a rubber band. Others like to fold down a corner of a denomination in a certain way or group them in their wallet by compartments. Others fold the whole bill in a variety of ways.

Here are a few possibilities you may want to try in your quest for the appropriate system for you. Ten dollar bills can be folded horizontally once, then vertically twice. Fives can be folded horizontally twice, and ones can be unfolded or rolled up in a rubber band. Any system that works for you is fine. (Adaptive aids catalogs also offer a "Talking Wallet," an expensive device that identifies bills by denomination.)

Coins are best identified by size, thickness, and ridges. Fifty cent pieces are the largest. Quarters are bigger than nickels and have ridges, whereas nickels are thicker and have smooth edges. Dimes and pennies are similar in size but dimes have ridges.

You may want to play a game to help you learn to efficiently retrieve dropped coins. Take a few coins and drop them onto a hard surface. Try to count how many you heard fall. The next time you accidentally drop your change, you will be able to tell how many coins are down and approximately where they are and what they are.

Another tip for helping to keep your money in order is to always ask for the kinds of denominations and coins you want. Before going to the bank, figure out the kinds of bills you want for that $50 withdrawal. Do you want three $10s, three $5s, four $1s, and four quarters, or some other combination? Planning ahead saves time and may result in helping you feel less stressed and rushed in the teller line.

Explain to the teller that you need time to fold and organize the bills as she hands them to you. As the teller counts out the bills, you may want to fold or band them on the spot. Take your time and do not allow yourself to be rushed. Make sure you put your money in your purse or wallet before you leave the teller window.

You also may want to make an appointment with your local bank to discuss the kinds of special services they offer to people with visual impairments. Ask about raised line or large print checks, and if they can arrange to do your personal banking at a desk rather than at a teller window to afford you more time and attention.

Paperwork, Paperwork

What about the rest of your paperwork? For example, do you need assistance with personal letters? You may need help to read your personal letters, but you certainly do not need help to answer them.

Your remaining vision may allow you to read letters with a magnifier or electronic aid. (See Chapter 9.) If your usable residual vision allows you to write with bold-line paper or a letter guide and felt pen—go for it! So what if your writing is so large that it takes you five pages to write one paragraph? That is just further evidence that you like to think BIG! Also remember that whether you have low vision or no vision, typing is always an option for writing letters. As an alternative, you can record your letters and encourage the correspondents in your life to tape theirs to you.

Okay, that wasn't so bad. But what about grocery lists, phone messages, and daily to-do lists? People handle grocery lists in many different ways. Some record them on cassette tape, item by item, as needed. Some people who have usable residual vision print their lists in large print. Others mark cans and boxes of food with index card labels written in large print, glue letters, or braille, or with talking labels, then file the label in a recipe box when they use up the can. When they go grocery shopping, they just check the recipe box for items they need.

You can write phone messages or to-do lists in large or bold print, in braille, or on a raised line drawing kit. You can also record them on a cassette or on your telephone answering machine tape.

> **Journal Note:** When I'm away from home and want to remind myself of something that's inconvenient to write down, I call home and leave the information as a message on my telephone answering machine.
>
> —*Vivian*

If you are a list-maker like we are, you are probably addicted to the darn things and we couldn't break you of the habit even if we wanted to. Actually, we recommend them. A daily to-do list can be just the thing to motivate you to get out of bed and out into the world. You can list one item or a dozen. If you don't accomplish everything today, there's always tomorrow. The value in the list is not to set the record for accomplishments, but to motivate you to organize your time and to show yourself that you really are getting things done. And you are—after all, you just completed reading this chapter, didn't you?

Organizational Checklist

- Sort your mail daily.

- Call billing companies to see if they will hold your mail temporarily. Ask if you can pay bills at local places of business.

- Experiment with bold-line paper, felt-tip pens, brighter lighting, tape recordings, and other adaptive aids so you can do correspondence independently.

- Practice writing your signature.

- Designate an assistant to work with you on your bills and mail, if needed. Set the ground rules at the first paper task session.

- File paid and unpaid bills in envelopes, boxes, or files.

- Develop your own folding system for money, and ask your bank about special services for visually impaired persons.

Adaptive Aids and Technology

We have taken a lot of time to inform you about the kinds of tasks you can do if you have the right tools. This is a good time to introduce you to some of the technology and adaptive aids that are available to help you accomplish your goals and achieve independence.

Throughout this chapter we list and suggest companies or organizations as referrals. Although we have worked successfully with those noted in the text and Appendixes, it is not our intention to promote one organization or company over another. We also recognize that technology changes rapidly and new adaptive aids and tools appear in the marketplace daily.

What are adaptive aids? They are devices and tools that enable visually impaired and other disabled people to perform tasks independently. An aid may be a new invention or an old tool that has been adapted with raised dots, braille, large print, or a voice simulator. Keep in mind, however, that aids are not cure-alls. They are simply one in an assortment of many options for performing daily tasks.

Aids are available in a variety of forms to fit almost any need. Some, such as prescriptive telescopic lenses and electronic travel aids, are prescribed by low vision specialists and/or ophthalmologists and require specialized training to use.

However, most aids are available without prescription or special training and can be purchased through adaptive aids catalogs (see the Appendix). Even better, many adaptive aids can be made at home by adapting your own appliances and tools with large print, raised lettering, or other marking methods to save you energy, patience, and time.

The Time of Day

Speaking of time, you may feel frustrated because you can no longer see the face of your watch and have to ask others for the time of day. This is unnecessary since adaptive watches and clocks are available in a myriad of styles.

There are watches with large print or with covers that open so you can feel the hands in relation to the raised dots, at five-minute increments. Other timers and clocks are marked with large print or raised dots. Talking models may be set to announce the time at set intervals or to sound an alarm at a specific time, for instance, as a wake-up signal or when medicine is to be taken.

Taking Your Medicine

Various aids offer new ways to monitor your health or administer medicine. Thermometers, devices to monitor blood pressure, pulse, and glucose, and scales are marked in large print or braille or announce the measurement in a synthesized voice.

Pill splitters divide pills into even halves, and liquid medication guides correctly measure teaspoon measurements. Diabetes-related devices measure insulin to preset levels and serve as needle guides. Many syringes are marked in large print.

In the Kitchen

Household adaptive aids are designed to ease your fears about cooking and carving and to make working in the kitchen safe.

These devices include a liquid level indicator that hooks over the lip of a cup and beeps or vibrates as the liquid nears the top of the cup, a one-cup beverage maker that heats liquids for soup or coffee, electromagnetic stoves that heat food without flames or heating elements, elbow-length oven mitts, vegetable slicing guides, and knife slicing guides.

Around the House

Other aids for the home include self-threading needles, sewing machine magnifiers, magnetic padlocks that require no combination and open with a magnetic sensor or with a combination of audible clicks, raised large print telephone dials, one-button automatic telephone dialing systems, and braille clothing tags.

Adaptive aids for the workshop or garage include rulers, yardsticks, and tape measures with raised, tactile readings or braille markings, saw guides with raised markings at specific degree points, drill guides, and squares, calipers, and micrometers with raised dot markings. Light probes and metal or voltage detectors locate light, flame, metal objects, or live electrical current with an audible signal.

Magnification Aids

You may want to use magnification aids so that you can maintain your household or job-related paperwork or pursue a favorite hobby. Magnifiers can help you read or see things that are fairly close to you, such as labels or reading material. They include hand-held devices, with or without illumination, such as circle or bar magnifiers that enlarge just one line of print, and page magnifiers that lie on and enlarge an entire page. Some are held in place a precise distance from the object or page by a stand, leaving your hands free. Many such magnifiers can magnify all or part of the newspaper, depending on the size of the newsprint.

Those whose vision requires stronger magnification may find that electronic magnifiers are helpful in accessing printed material. These include closed circuit television (CCTV) systems that can magnify an object or page 60 times normal size. The system includes a camera and a zoom lens that photograph and enlarge the object, then display it on a television monitor. Small, portable models are available for use away from home, and some can be connected to a computer.

If you lack any significant usable vision, magnification aids may not be of help and you may want to try to use reading machines. The Optacon, an electronic reading device, translates print into vibrating letter configurations that you read with your fingertip. You scan a line of print with a small camera that you hold in one hand. The index finger of your other hand rests on a tactile array of vibrating pins that form print letters you recognize with your fingertip. Use of the Optacon requires specialized and intensive training.

Talking Devices

Another reading machine is the Kurzweil Personal Reader. This talking device uses a computer-controlled camera to scan lines of print. You place the page of print in a scanner and the text is read aloud via a voice synthesizer. Other scanning devices, offered by companies such as Telesensory Systems and Hewlett Packard, are optical character readers that scan text and convert it to a computer file. The computer reads the text aloud through a voice synthesizer or displays it as a braille display.

Many magazines, newspapers, and books are available through your local library in large print or braille, or on tape. Four-track tape players and Talking Book machines are required to play the four-track tapes and flexible discs that the National Library Service offers. These machines are provided free of cost to legally blind and physically disabled persons.

Commercially offered cassette tapes may be available in compressed speech or accelerated speech versions. Compressed speech uses speech in which either portions of the pauses between words have been deleted or shortened vowel sounds are used. The material is re-recorded in the shorter version and the sound of the speech is not affected.

Accelerated speech is text that is recorded at normal speed, but reproduced and played at an accelerated speed. Highly accelerated speech may produce an annoying distortion of the sound of the voice, but many cassette players have pitch controlling options that counteract this problem.

Aids to Writing

Those of you with some usable residual vision who feel confident with your printing or handwriting skills may accomplish writing and communication chores with aids designed specifically for these tasks. Script writing guides are templates with an opening that corresponds to either one line of space or to a full page on a sheet of paper. Many designs include adaptations for drawing vertical lines or for use on nonstandard size paper.

Other templates are designed to enable you to address envelopes, fill in checks, or sign your name. They are made from metal, plastic, or cardboard, and have windows that correspond to the type of document you are working with. Many adaptive aids catalogs can make templates to suit your particular needs or documents.

If you have some usable residual vision, bold-line paper may be helpful. Bold-line paper is writing paper with heavy, dark lines in place of the standard light blue ones. When used with a thick-tipped felt pen, these two aids may be all you need to be able to write independently.

Those of you who have touch-typing skills need to temporarily mark the home reference keys, F and J, so you can continue writing. Be sure to check your margins and ribbon control before typing. You can set your margins by measuring the distance in finger-widths. Attach a tab of masking tape at the lower right edge of the backing page to alert you that you are near the end of the page.

You also may want to investigate computer options. Recent inventions and innovations in peripherals (add-on options) and software programs make computers very accessible to people who are losing, or have lost, their sight.

Those of you who learn braille may use a slate and stylus, a small, portable template, and device for writing braille. This method is akin to writing with a pencil and paper. As a faster method of writing letters and notes, you may want to use a Perkins braille writer, a keyed device used for writing braille.

User Friendly Computers

Large print computers or those linked to CCTV systems are accessible to low vision users. Other options allow users to enter information through a standard or braille keyboard and retrieve information in braille, in print, or through speech synthesizers. Print scanners linked to a computer can read the material and send it to a computer file where it can be read by a synthetic voice. Special options allow you to translate text from braille to print and vice versa. Printers can produce the text in either braille or print. Spell checking software options proofread your text and allow you to correct your mistakes.

> **Journal Note:** Since I have now lost just about all of my vision and cannot read the computer monitor visually, my employer is buying a device so that I will have access to my computer monitor through synthetic speech.
>
> —*Susan*

For those who learn braille, paperless braille (also called Versabraille) stores information on disks and is read with the fingertips on a tactile display. You can use the system to create your own braille text, edit it, and interface with typewriters and computers.

> **Journal Note:** I am a teacher for the blind. I work with children who are blind and handicapped. Depending on my job duties, I use a variety of adaptive aids in the classroom. I use braille and standard type-writers, a closed circuit television, a computer with a braille printer, and a human classroom aide who is on the school staff. In addition to teaching academics, I teach my students daily living skills.
>
> *—Julia*

> **Journal Note:** I am presently attending a junior col-lege. I use prerecorded textbooks and a reader for class reading requirements. I use a personal computer with a speech output in order to write papers and complete homework assignments. I often hire my college readers to assist me with personal and paper-related tasks.
>
> *—Michael*

Working with Pictures

You say you don't deal in words as much as in drawings or pic-tures? Why not give the raised line drawing kit a try? The kit uses a pen-like stylus to form letters or drawings on special Mylar sheets that cover a drawing board. The drawn lines are visible and you can trace them with your fingers. This kit is best used on a temporary basis because the drawings are legible, but not of high quality. A similar device, a dot inverter, makes embossed dots on a sheet of paper, allowing you to form simple maps or figures.

Thermoform is another possibility for those who work with pictures or raised figures. The thermoform system uses an oven to heat plastic sheets. The heated sheets can be embossed with lines, dots, or raised letters. You can glue braille dots, yarn, string, beads, or any three-dimensional material onto a page and thermoform it to make pictures, diagrams, coloring books, etc. Thermoform sheets are also used to duplicate braille pages from a master sheet.

Making Your Own Aids

You may want to create your own adaptive aids by marking or labeling them yourself. You can easily mark the controls on your microwave oven or the outside of a measuring cup with markings made with glue or fluorescent Hi-Marks. These items dry into easily seen, hardened letters or dots. Label makers make braille, raised print, large print, or talking labels that can be attached to just about anything. Other labeling methods include glue letters on a 3 x 5 inch card or cut-out cardboard letters.

Outside the Home

You may require additional aids outside the home. These may include bioptics or telescopes, which allow you to see print or objects at some distance. They may even allow you to continue driving. Telescopes are prescribed and may be incorporated into your eyeglass lenses, swung down from an arm on your frames, or clipped on as needed. Telescopes may enable you to see the classroom blackboard, locate and read street and store signs, read bus and house numbers, view a baseball game, or locate birds in trees, see the pins in a bowling alley, watch children in another room or at the playground, and locate the newspaper delivered to your yard.

Travel aids allow you to move safely and independently in your environment. These include rigid or folding long white canes, dog guides, and electronic travel aids.

Cane use is taught by a trainer of orientation and mobility

techniques who determines the proper cane length for each individual and teaches techniques for detecting and traveling around objects along travel routes.

> **Journal Note:** Thanks to the Department of Rehabilitation, I feel very comfortable traveling using a white cane. I go to Senior Citizen outings, to the Braille Transcription Project, to visit friends, and to accomplish logistical activities, such as banking, for example.
>
> *—Janice*

> **Journal Note:** Even though I have traveled with dog guides before, I prefer using a cane. I feel very competent in my traveling abilities. I feel that people who use their dog guides as a means of traveling are usually insecure about their traveling abilities and a dog guide would aid them in crossing complex intersections.
>
> *—Ray*

Dog guide training and travel instruction are provided by several dog guide schools for the blind throughout the United States. Dogs used for travel assistance by the visually impaired are correctly termed *dog guides*, not *seeing eye dog, guide dog,* or *leader dog,* as these are copyrighted terms held by their respective dog guide schools. Good cane traveling skills are a prerequisite to dog guide training.

> **Journal Note:** I have used both a cane and a dog guide for safe travel. Although I have sufficient cane skills to get around, a dog guide allows me to travel at a fast pace—about four miles an hour.
>
> *—Michael*

> **Journal Note:** The reason that I have chosen a dog guide over a white cane is easy. The dog guide offers

me the freedom I never ever had before, security, and, by all means, the chance to not feel that I'm talking to thin air. Having a dog guide has given me the chance to give myself a life that was never available with the white cane. When you're using a white cane, you have to work and work and work and stumble and stumble and stumble. For myself, I would take a dog guide over a white cane any day.

—Alice

Electronic travel aids include the laser cane, the Pathsounder, the Sonic Guide, and the Mowat Sensor, all of which are prescribed and require specialized training to use. These aids send out light beams or ultrasound waves that come into contact with objects in their path. The device vibrates or emits a sound when the beam or wave hits an object. The Night Vision Aid, a prescribed, hand-held illumination aid, improves vision at night by amplifying available light.

Orientation aids familiarize you with the layout of a particular building or site. These include tactile or three-dimensional maps, models, and verbal recordings of site descriptions or travel routes. Some cities offer tactile maps for visually impaired citizens and many public facilities, such as airports, provide models or recorded site descriptions. (Many airlines also offer flight information, including descriptions about the inside of their planes, in braille.)

Adaptive Aid Costs

You may already be adding up the cost of these items in your mind and thinking twice about benefit versus cost. Most adaptive aids are relatively inexpensive and some are free. For example, nonoptical aids or environmental aids that are part of the home or work place often cost nothing to implement.

Nonoptical aids improve the environment rather than alter the things you are looking at. They include illumination, light transmission, reflection control, and contrast.

According to your needs, brighter or dimmer room lighting may improve your home or office illumination. Experiment with window coverings, incandescent and fluorescent light, and the benefits of standing versus flexible arm lamps.

Prescriptive lenses, filters, or absorptive lenses incorporated into your own prescription lenses, and the use of non-glare paper or a sheet of yellow acetate placed over a page of print may reduce glare and highlight contrast to improve light transmission when reading or writing. Visors, sideshields, and specially treated lenses may reduce reflection.

Contrast can maximize the use of whatever amount of vision you have. Light plates on a dark tablecloth, dark tools hung on a white board, a light doorknob on a dark door, and fluorescent strips on stair risers can make things previously unnoticed sharpen into view.

Where Do I Begin?

Pretty overwhelming, isn't it? It is hard to know where to begin to select items. You may want to start slowly by trying out some adaptive aids before buying. Contact agencies serving the blind, rehabilitation facilities for the visually impaired, and college disabled student programs and ask if they offer free access to adaptive aids.

The decision to use or not to use an adaptive aid is based on the amount of time that you will spend using it versus its cost. These two factors should balance each other so that the time you spend is worth the cost. For example, it may take you an hour to read five pages of print using a CCTV that may cost over $1,000. Only you can decide if that is a good balance for you.

You should also consider the amount of residual vision you have, and its efficiency, when deciding on an adaptive aid. Although you may have some residual vision, it may not be usable or efficient enough to use effectively with an adaptive aid. You may see well enough to write legibly on bold-line paper, but not see well enough to read your handwriting. It may be more beneficial and practical for you to learn to read braille to perform your paper-related tasks.

Once you have tried out some devices, you may want to obtain an adaptive aids catalog. As you go through the catalog, look over the list you made in Chapter 3, the one that outlines the tasks you can do with an adaptive aid. Then choose items according to your own priorities and needs. You will find that, as you get used to using something as basic as bold-line paper or a signature guide, your confidence will grow and allow you to try more sophisticated tools. In no time at all, you may find yourself perusing computer catalogs!

Where can you get information about companies and products that fit your needs? First, you can recontact the agencies for blindness and visual impairment that you first called for information on vision loss. **The American Foundation for the Blind**, the **American Council for the Blind**, the **National Federation of the Blind**, the **National Association of Visually Handicapped** and the **National Society to Prevent Blindness**, listed in Chapter 3 (and information in the Appendices) can provide you with information and referrals regarding your needs.

Those with low vision may want to try a low vision clinic that will introduce them to low vision devices. There are over 250 low vision clinics, agencies, or programs in the United States. Your doctor or ophthalmologist should be able to refer you to one in your area. If not, call a local, county, or state agency that serves visually impaired persons or call the **American Foundation for the Blind**, which has a listing of low vision clinics.

State rehabilitation and vocational services also provide introduction to and training with adaptive aids as part of their program. Look in the phone book for the State Department of Rehabilitation, the Commission for the Blind, or Services for the Blind. The name of the agency that offers rehabilitation services varies from state to state.

If you know what type of product you want, but do not know the manufacturer or the product name, **ABLEDATA** may be able to help you. ABLEDATA is a database service that lists and describes products for people with disabilities. Its product descriptions list the generic name, manufacturer, brand name, availability, cost, and product description. ABLEDATA charges a small fee, but searches up to eight pages are free. Write or call:

> ABLEDATA, Adaptive Equipment Center,
> Newington Children's Hospital
> 181 East Cedar Street, Newington, CT 06111
> (800) 344-5405.

If you want to contact a company directly, call and ask for information on products designed for use by visually impaired persons. A limited list of companies that manufacture technology for blind and visually impaired users is listed in the Appendices.

Take some time to investigate adaptive aids and technology. They offer you the possibility of regaining independence in virtually all aspects of your life.

Organizational Checklist

- Contact an agency for the blind and visually impaired about adaptive aids and technology.
- Call your State Department of Rehabilitation or Commission for the Blind to ask for adaptive aids information and training.
- Ask your doctor to refer you to a low vision clinic, or contact the American Foundation for the Blind (AFB) for a low vision program in your area, if applicable.
- Call or write ABLEDATA at (800) 344-5405 for product information.
- Call a vendor or company directly for specific information on its products.

10

Becoming Socially Active Again

The more impaired your vision becomes, the less you may feel a part of the sighted world. Vision is a major source of information gathering and without it you are cut off from a lot of clues you once unconsciously depended on. Where you were once able to see a friend's facial expression, you may now be able to see only his shadow. He may eventually become a disembodied voice.

You also may feel detached from your own body. You may wonder what your face is doing or what emotions it is expressing. You may even feel faceless. It is common to find yourself losing interest in your appearance because you cannot see the results and use other people's visual reactions to you as a mirror. In fact, you may have stopped thinking about yourself in visual terms altogether.

How do you deal with these problems and start becoming reoriented to the world? One way to begin is by accepting that it can be a lengthy process. You do not decide to become reoriented one day and achieve it the next. People who are especially visual find the process extremely difficult and some never fully adjust.

You can, however, take steps to help the process along by getting out into the sighted world and functioning in the best way you can. You may make mistakes and you may be embarrassed. You may want to quit and live the life of a hermit. But you may also surprise yourself with your strength, perseverance, and humor.

At first, your family and friends may be the key to helping you stay in touch with the sighted world. Invite them into your life. Your preparations need not be elaborate and you need not feel that you have to function as the perfect host. Plan something specific at first. Ask a friend over to watch television—and you can serve canned juice and potato chips. Invite a relative to join you in listening to a radio program. Ask the teenager in your life to read the comics in the daily newspaper to you. Have your children take turns walking with you to the corner each evening until you feel safe and confident traveling alone. The possibilities are endless.

Try to restore some normalcy to your life. If you have cooked Sunday family dinners for fifteen years, blindness should not stop this tradition. You may not be able to serve the usual roast beef and mashed potatoes (yet) but you can enjoy the family gathering over a meal. You can call family members and say, "We're having a change of menu. I'm serving pizza and soda this week—and by the way, can you pick up the pizza on your way over?" Serve that double cheese and anchovy deluxe on paper plates and drink your soda from cans until you have mastered pouring. By doing this, you are showing your family that the food is not the important thing. *They* are. You are telling them that you want to continue traveling in the mainstream of life—with them.

> **Journal Note:** I enjoy entertaining in my home. I feel that the key to a successful party is to plan ahead and be organized. I recently had twenty-five relatives over to enjoy the holidays.
>
> —*Rachael*

Fun and Games

Games are also a great way to spend time with friends and many can be played without the use of vision. The following is a sampling of games for which you do not require vision or which are easily adaptable. They are available at most toy stores or can be ordered from an adaptive aids catalog.

Think Tic Tac Toe	Topple
Stuff It	Perfection
Aggravation	Twenty Questions
Simon	Clash
Cootie	Ungame
Trivial Pursuit	Hi-Q
Jeopardy	Othello
Scruples	Monopoly
Operation	Scrabble
Twister	Playing Cards
Password	Checkers

Journal Note: My children enjoy playing table games. I adapted the Uno cards with braille and my husband used glue to mark the lines in the game Sorry. Now we can all play these games together.

—Emily

Many other games can be adapted for play by adding glue letters or dots. For instance, chess enthusiasts can continue their matches after marking the top of each black piece with a glue dot. The shape of the piece will distinguish a knight from a pawn. Consult an adaptive aids catalog if you are a poker player or a fan of some other game that requires special adaptation. Many offer a wide variety of adaptive cards and games that may be played by both sighted and blind people.

Journal Note: For a long period of time I was afraid to play games because I thought I wouldn't be able to keep up with my sighted friends. So instead of using games as a bridge, I used them as a wall. Luckily, my friends were sensitive to this and let me know that it's alright if it takes me a couple of minutes to figure a word in Scrabble or a hand in poker. As a result, I've become a good game player. In fact, my friends now accuse me of playing with "marked cards!"

—Vivian

Whatever you do together, feel free to discuss your vision and to express yourself in visual words. Voice your fears and concerns, and encourage your loved ones to express theirs as well. They may be waiting for you to bring up the subject and may sigh in relief when you do.

Out and About

By now, even if you consider yourself a homebody, you may be feeling a touch of cabin fever. If outings to the beach, church, amusement parks, rock concerts, or art exhibits were once a part of your life, there is no reason why they should not continue to be.

Journal Note: I feel that blindness should not get in the way of doing anything you want to do. Some time ago, I went to a ski resort and had a great time with the support of friends and the aid of the ski instructor. He guided me by clicking two short, shallow, bamboo sticks about 25 to 50 feet ahead of me and I was able to independently ski down an intermediate slope.

—Janice

Journal Note: Although I am seventy years old, I am the kind of person who enjoys getting about. I participate in a gym class for the disabled and am taking an introductory class in theater at a nearby junior college.

I enjoy reading books on flexible disc, tape, and braille. If a college course book is not on tape, I can use a human reader in order to get my assignments done. During the dinner hour and on special occasions, I enjoy playing the piano for people in the retirement center where I reside. I enjoy living around other people and interacting with them. I believe in living life to the fullest.

—*Rose*

Call your favorite museum, zoo, theater, or gallery a few days before you visit and ask about programs for the blind or disabled. Many places offer guided tours or lectures especially designed for visually impaired patrons. Ask about the busiest hours and plan accordingly. Plan to arrive early for a scheduled event such as a concert or play. This way you can take care of your needs and avoid the rush of last-minute crowds.

If you require the driving services of a friend or relative, apply to the Department of Motor Vehicles for a parking placard for the disabled. This allows your driver to park in spaces reserved for the disabled, in metered zones without paying, and in green zones without time restrictions.

Always carry something to identify you as visually impaired. It may be a special transit pass, an emergency medical card, a medical alert bracelet, or a homemade card that describes your vision loss. Those of you who go through a rehabilitation program will most likely have a rigid or folding long white cane, optical aids, or a dog guide to help alert others to your blindness.

It is often helpful to take a cassette tape recorder on any outing. It can serve as your camera by recording the mood of the day in sound. Take along some music cassettes and you can listen to music while traveling or waiting. Those with some usable residual vision can take a simple, aim-and-shoot model camera and save your memories as photographs. You may also want to bring along a puzzle, game, knitting, a book in large print, braille, or on tape, or some other entertaining item.

While riding in the car, remember that half the fun is getting there. Those of you with partial sight should take an interest in the scenery as you travel and comment on what you can see. Observations such as, "Gosh, there's a balloon trailing out the window of that camper," "I see we're going through some trees," or "It's so clear I can see the outline of the mountains today," may make the ride more interesting for you and will inform your companion about what you can see.

Feel free to ask your sighted friend to describe the scenery. Ask specific questions about the clouds in the sky, the colors of the leaves, or even the antics of the drivers around you. Some days taking notice of what you can and cannot see may be depressing. If this is the case, concentrate on a more positive subject for your conversation, listen to a tape you can both enjoy, or play an individualized game such as Hi-Q.

Upon arrival at your destination, locate the restroom facilities, water fountains, food concessions, and exits. Unfamiliar public restrooms offer a special challenge. When you enter a strange restroom, stop and look for the light source. The light in combination with exploring the perimeters of the room may be all you need to quickly orient yourself to this restroom. A cane or an arm sweep may be helpful in locating wastebaskets, hand blowers, and sinks.

If you are separated while your companion gets tickets or food, ask him to find you a seat in a well-traveled spot. If for any reason you become lost or separated in a crowd, find a seat and wait for your friend, or ask the first person you encounter to help you locate the information or ticket booth.

Remember that you can still enjoy the same social and recreational activities you always have. You just may have to develop new strategies to make up for your loss of vision.

> **Journal Note:** I am the coordinator of a local bowling league for the blind. I encourage bowlers to orient themselves to the center by pacing or squaring off from the ball return unit. I am also the coordinator of

the Bay Area USA Blind Athletes Association. Each year blind children and adults are encouraged to participate in swimming and track and field events. Participants are grouped by their age and degree of blindness. Short tubes or guide ropes are available for those who choose to use them.

—John

The following excursions to a zoo, a museum, and a party are described from the perspectives of people with both progressive and sudden vision loss. They may help you form your own strategies for enjoying visual entertainment.

It's a Jungle Out There

Once you have entered the zoo, you may feel overwhelmed by the sights, sounds, and smells of the place. Before setting off for a tour, sit down and take a few moments to get your bearings. Use this time to notice the bright colors of a welcoming banner, to isolate the sound of a baby cooing as a stroller glides by, or to catch the unmistakable scent of the monkeys brought by on the breeze. Take time to talk about which animals you would like to see first and participate in the decisions to be made.

Those with some vision should start with the larger animals. Elephants, rhinos, and giraffes are often good subjects. Even if the elephant is not close enough or is located in poor lighting, you may be able to discern its movement or hear its trumpeting. If a trainer or feeder is nearby, ask questions. Facts about the animal's size, weight, diet, or habits can help give you a better "picture" of it.

Many zoos equip the exhibits or cages with "talking boxes" that play recorded information about the animals. You may want to record on your tape that you discovered how to tell the African elephants from the Indian elephants or the crocodiles from the alligators. If you use your camera, you will also have a visual record.

Feed the animals, if allowed. When the seal nips a fish from your fingers, you will not only be able to view it at close range, you will also feel its whiskers brush your hand and smell its salty (not to mention fishy) breath.

A trip to the petting zoo can also be fun. Before you enter, talk to your friend about any special needs you may have here. The animals often are allowed to roam about freely, so you may want to be warned about sudden movements. Ask your friend to tell you when an animal is near and to place your hand on it. This way you will be able to pat the goat's head without first discovering its horns. Ask your friend to guide you clear of animal paws, hooves, and droppings.

A guided tram tour may be a comfortable way for you to see the zoo. Although you may not be able to see everything from your seat, the information given by the guide is usually interesting and entertaining. Those of you who want to use your tape recorder as a camera can return, time and again, to the lion's cage in the comfort of your own easy chair.

When you are ready for a break, try to find a spot with a variety of sights and sounds. A waterfall, a children's playground, a duck pond, or a carousel all provide pleasant background noises and views as you relax and refresh. Try to find a place with bright visual scenery as well, or a shady spot if that fits your needs best.

But Is It Art?

Do a little homework before you visit a museum, and find out about what you are going to see. If it is a new or traveling exhibit, ask the museum to send you some promotional material about it. Get books or tapes about the artist and his or her work from your local library or the National Library Service for the Blind and Physically Handicapped. If necessary, ask a friend to read to you and to describe the pictures of the works of art.

Once in the museum, look at the building itself as a work of art. Those with usable residual vision should visually note the lighting, the period of architecture, and the style of exhibitry. If necessary, ask your friend about the height of the ceiling, the color of the walls, and the curve of the doorways. Touch the carving on the pillars or columns, feel the plushness of the carpet underfoot, and take note of the silence of the room.

Ask an administrator for a taped tour or if a docent could accompany you. If the exhibit is sculptural, ask if you can touch the works.

When you are looking at the painting or sculpture, ask your friend to describe it to you. Those with usable residual vision should use their visual aids to observe the piece.

Think out loud a bit. When you say, "I remember that apple on the derby as being bright green. Am I right?" or "I wonder why the artist placed a melting watch on the rock!" you'll be enjoying the visual exhibit a new way and letting your friend know what you are picturing.

Docents are usually happy to answer questions about the artist or his style, so do not hesitate to ask about something that interests or puzzles you. Keep your cassette recorder on to capture all of the conversations, or take photographs if possible. Later you will be able to share the exhibit with your friends or loved ones.

Party Time

An invitation to a party or a large family gathering may trigger conflicting emotions. Although you may look forward to the social aspects of the party, you may be worried about how you will function there. Perhaps you are concerned that you will be left alone for hours or that your friends will feel "stuck" with you. Or maybe you are uncertain about how to mix and mingle with the other guests. However, with a little planning, you can deal with these situations and begin to treasure each new invitation.

R.S.V.P.

When you call to accept, ask your host some questions to help you prepare for the party. Find out who will be invited and some background information about each guest. Maybe one of the guests does the same type of work you do or has a similar hobby. At the party you will be able to seek out this person, knowing you have something in common.

Food is a highlight of any party, so ask about the menu. Do the refreshments sound like something you can easily handle? Will there be finger food or will some cutting be required?

Ask if there will be any special entertainment. If nothing formal is planned, you may want to come prepared. Look over your cassette music tapes or photos and choose a few to take with you.

Finally, ask permission to arrive a bit early to get the "lay of the land." You will want time to find the bathroom, locate the stairs, and uncover any hazards, such as low-hanging plants or a child's rocking horse out in the open.

Can I Bring Anything?

Even if a program of entertainment is planned, it is still a good idea to bring along some of your own. Your cassette recorder can be used to tape conversations you have with other guests. You may bring a group game or activity, such as Trivial Pursuit or *The Book of Questions*. In order to assure that you can individually participate in table games, bring an adaptive game for everyone to enjoy, such as a deck of adaptive playing cards.

Consider bringing an object that might serve as an icebreaker. Perhaps you could choose a beautiful Japanese fan, a family photo album, some vintage music tapes, or some balloons to blow up and pass around. These can be used to draw people into conversation with you.

Journal Note: When I attended a new church for the first time I brought along my portable braille computer as a conversation piece. I really didn't need it to take notes since my cassette recorder or slate and stylus (a device equivalent to paper and pencil) would have worked just as well. However, I guessed that curiosity about the machine would help people feel more comfortable talking with me. It proved to be a great icebreaker and I met several people as a result.

—Vivian

If the planned menu includes food that you cannot easily handle and eat, for personal or medical reasons, take along an item you can contribute to the gathering. You might want to bring fried chicken, fruit salad, a lemon cake—anything that might be enjoyed by all.

Come In and Join the Party

When you arrive at the party, ask your host to show you around a bit. Find the bathroom, the refreshment table, and the cooking or barbecue area. Ask the host to point out steps, hanging plants, or other hazards. You may want to request that he introduce you to the other guests and that he verbally or visually check up on you every half hour if possible. One of the greatest concerns about parties is the fear of being left alone. Nobody wants to be a wallflower. A good way to avoid this is to find a seat near the refreshments. People tend to naturally gravitate to food, so you will have a steady flow of conversationalists to choose from.

But how do you strike up a conversation? Chances are it will be just as easy or difficult as it was before you lost your sight. Although you may have depended on eye contact as an opener in the past, you can now learn to use other methods. If someone is sitting next to you, assume that they want to talk to you (after all, this is a party, right?). Introduce yourself and extend your hand immediately. This is an assertive, nonverbal gesture that gives you the opportunity to get a better mental picture of your new friend. From his handshake you can get an idea of his height, weight, degree of nervousness, and whether his work is done indoors or out.

Unless you are a palm reader, you probably won't be able to tell his astrological sign, so you will have to ask. When you do ask, try to look in the direction of his face, or at least turn your head or body in his direction. Ask open-ended questions or suggest that he describe what is going on around you. His version of John's belly flop into the pool or Jane's snubbing of Harry's advances can be a welcome alternative to small talk and make you feel more a part of the action.

If you feel ready for a snack and want to try the party fare, get your new acquaintance's opinion about what looks inviting. If the food is served on paper plates, use two or more to provide extra support. While your friend is serving himself, you may want to ask him to serve you, too. You can ask him to tell you where he is placing the food on your plate in relation to a clock. Ask what is at 12 o'clock, 3 o'clock, and so on. Also ask him to point out foods that are particularly drippy.

If you would like to serve yourself, place your plate as close to the serving dish as possible. Locate the serving utensil by trailing your fingers around the outside rim of the serving dish. If the utensil has slipped down into the dish, ask someone to show you where it is. The type of utensil—tongs, spoon, or spatula—will give you clues about what type of food is in the dish and how to move the food to your plate. By serving yourself, you will automatically know where the item is on your plate.

To pour a cold beverage, hook your index finger over the lip of the cup up to the first knuckle. Stop pouring when the liquid touches the bottom of your finger.

When you are ready to cut your food, first explore the size and shape of the plate with one of your utensils. Use your fork to measure off a bite-size piece, then slide your knife down the back of the fork until it touches the food item. Cut along the back edge of the fork until the cut piece is free.

If the setting is informal and you must balance your plate on your lap, you may feel more comfortable cutting your food at a counter or on a table before settling down to eat. Keep your cup or glass under your seat to avoid tipping it. In a more formal dinner setting, use your chair as a reference to help you locate your place setting. Make a quick check to note how close together the table settings are to one another and to find the location of your glass or cup so you can avoid spills.

If you are worried about spills or dribbles, tuck your napkin or a paper towel in at your collar. As anyone who has ever eaten lobster in a restaurant knows, there is nothing embarrassing or inappropriate about wearing a bib.

If you sense that your friend is getting ready to move on, be sure to ask him to tell you when he leaves. Then you won't find yourself commenting on the bean dip to an empty chair. When you are temporarily left alone, focus on various conversations and faces around you. This opportunity will allow you to decide who you may want to visit with next. You may take this opportunity to visually take note of the decorations, the clothing, or costumes of the guests, and the decor of the room.

When your host or hostess checks back with you, ask him or her to introduce you to someone you want to meet. Maybe you heard the name "Ziggy" in passing and would like to meet the person who matches the moniker. Perhaps you are feeling really brave and decide to talk to the first person with whom you come in contact.

> **Journal Note:** When we have a party or a gathering at our home, we make sure to prepare the food items well in advance. We discuss and determine how the furniture should be arranged to accommodate our and our guests' visual needs. Our family enjoys going to movies and sports activities. I took my boys fishing recently and we had a great time.
>
> —*John*

Being a Good Host

As a host, there is a great deal you can do to make your visually impaired guest feel comfortable. Others will look to you as an
example of how to interact with him. Introduce your friend to the
other guests and get a conversation going before you leave. Then
check up on him later to see how he is doing. Suggest a seat in a
busy place near the food, record player, or entertainment. When
planning the menu, keep your friend in mind. If you are unsure
about the types of food to serve your visually impaired guest, call
and ask him.

Stay in Touch

Although you may not get out of the house much at first, there
are many ways to stay in touch with the sighted world. Use the
media to keep you informed and entertained. When you watch
TV with a friend, ask her to describe what the actors are wearing.
Questions like "Are bow ties popular again?" and "Just how
short is that miniskirt?" will clue her in to your interests. Question
her about hairstyles and current fashionable lengths. This will
keep you abreast of current styles and designs.

Most television shows also reflect changes in home styles and
furnishings. Inquire about the hound's-tooth pattern on the chair
or the colors in the Tiffany lamp shade in the living room of your
favorite sitcom.

Many of the laughs on TV depend on silent sight gags or
physical gestures. Ask your friend to describe or reenact what
happened during the pause.

Television descriptive services, such as **Descriptive Video
Service** and **Washington Ear** provide narration describing visual features of dramatic television programs, including costuming,
lighting, and physical action. The service uses a separate channel
accessible through an adapter that is compatible with standard
television and video cassette recorders. To reach either service
write or call:

Descriptive Video Service
WGBH-TV
125 Western Avenue
Boston, MA 02134
(617) 492-2777

Washington Ear, Inc.
35 University Boulevard East
Silver Spring, MD 20901
(301) 681-6636

During the Break

When it is time for a station break, take note of the commercials. They can alert you to new products, foods, or packaging that may simplify your life. These new items also mirror the public's needs and can give you insights into changes within society.

The Movies

Those of you who are ready for the bigger picture can butter some popcorn, load up on Raisinettes, and take in a movie. Films are equally conducive to keeping you up-to-date and have the advantage of presenting a much larger image. Those with some usable vision may be able to see some of the film if you position yourself appropriately to your needs. When you go to a movie with a friend, ask him or her to automatically explain the silent action or to fill you in only when you request it.

Talking Tomes

Those of you who thought you would have to give up *Newsweek* or *Time*, take heart. Magazines and books are available through the **National Library Service for the Blind and Physically Handicapped**. They provide talking book machines that play hard and flexible discs, four-track tape players and tapes, and braille books. Catalogs are available on flexible disk, in braille, and in large print. Most of the materials and machines are provided without charge and are great resources for education and entertainment. **Recording for the Blind** records and lends textbooks to blind and physically or perceptually disabled persons and is useful for those pursuing educational, personal, or professional research.

On the Radio

Radio Information Services provide radio channels and programs that contain news and information on community events. The services are broadcast on open, freely accessible channels or on closed channels that require a reception box available through the broadcasting station. State radio services are often listed in the telephone book under **Radio Reading Service**, **Radio Talking Book**, or **Radio Information Service**. Call (813) 974-4193 for the phone number in your state. (See Appendix.)

The Human Factor

Your sighted friends and relatives also can be a means of obtaining information about trends, fads, and fashions. If dressing fashionably is important to you, ask a fashion-conscious friend to advise you on an outfit. See if the teenager in your life can help you update your look by putting pieces of your wardrobe together in new ways. Use what you have learned from the media to ask questions. You could say, "I saw on 'L.A. Law' that the men were wearing suspenders. Would they look good with my gray suit?" or "*McCall's* says to accessorize with scarves this fall. Can you help me choose one for my green blouse?"

Perhaps you would prefer some professional advice. Most large department stores now offer personalized shopper service. Personalized shoppers are store employees who can help you select and coordinate your clothing. Call your local store to make an appointment, or shop during the quiet hours when a salesperson can give you more time and attention.

Make Every Contact Count

With a little imagination, you can use just about anything or anyone as a link to the sighted world. A conversation with the paper boy could expose you to the latest slang expression. A television commercial could alert you to free medical services. A trip to the grocery store may reveal new trends in gourmet foods. Even though escargot-on-a-stick may not be your cup of tea, you will have uncovered something new. Each new discovery is one more step toward moving successfully in the sighted world.

Organizational Checklist

Home
- Review the board games or puzzles in the house. Place those that require little or no vision in an easily accessible spot. Adapt others with glue dots or braille, and record instructions and printed sections on a cassette tape.
- Contact the National Library Service for talking book machines, flexible discs, tapes, tape players, records, and so on.
- Call local museums, theaters, zoos, and galleries, and ask about programs for the blind or disabled.
- Apply to the Department of Motor Vehicles for a parking placard for the disabled.

- Gather together a cassette player, blank tapes, individualized games, an easy-to-operate camera, folding cane, optical aids, and so on, and store them in a travel bag or backpack.

- Place an ID card that notes your degree of visual impairment, a transit pass, an emergency medical card, or a homemade 3 x 5 inch card in your purse or wallet.

Party-Goer

- Call the party host ahead of time and ask about the guests, food, and entertainment. Ask permission to arrive early.

- Take the packed backpack to the party.

- Pack a snack to eat or share.

- Take along a puzzle or game to share.

Host

- Give the visually impaired guest a tour. Point out the bathroom, refreshment area, entertainment area, and any hazards such as stairs or low-hanging plants.

- Suggest a seat near the food, record player, or entertainment.

- Introduce your visually impaired guest to other guests and get a conversation going before leaving the group.

- Visually or verbally check in with your visually impaired guest, for support purposes, once in a while.

11

Handling Embarrassing Situations

Whether your sight loss is sudden or progressive, you will probably soon realize that the public has a lot to learn about the visually impaired. Most people think that being blind means having no sight at all—living in total darkness, irreversible blackness. If you use a cane or dog guide, people may automatically assume that you have no vision, rather than limited vision.

The public often assumes that you have limited abilities that restrict your ability to perform all the everyday activities of life. They may see you as unemployable, asocial, asexual, depressing, or pitiable. Worse yet, they may put you up on a pedestal and see you as courageous, admirable, and in possession of superhuman hearing or over-heightened senses. But in reality, you are just you—as you have always been—except for some loss of sight.

Because of so many public misconceptions about blindness, you may at times have to work harder to get others to see you as a capable, normal human being who happens to be visually impaired. You may need to become verbally assertive because you cannot depend on visual clues to break the ice.

At first you may not want anyone to know that you are losing your sight. You may be afraid they will assume that you are helpless or mentally deficient. You may feel that you are constantly on display and that those who love you are watching your every move. Therefore, you may begin to view your blindness as embarrassing. Guess what? You are buying into the public's perception of blindness. You will have to change your attitude so that you can guide others to respond more favorably to you.

Your Mind's Eye

You can begin by looking at your eyes and their assistive aids in new ways. The look of your eyes may have changed during the course of your vision loss. Perhaps your eyes appear sunken or scarred. Maybe one or both of your eyes move or scan the field of vision in a distracting, involuntary way. You may be wearing an artificial eye and feel uncomfortable about its appearance. You may even be afraid that others are repulsed by the way your eyes look.

Those of you who feel that your eyes are unattractive or distracting may want to consider wearing dark glasses to avoid embarrassment for you and for those you meet. If you wear a prosthetic eye, you may take comfort in knowing that they are practically undetectable from the real thing. As Tom Sullivan tells in his book, *If You Could See What I Hear*, his false eyes are much more attractive than his natural ones ever were.

> **Journal Note:** Because my left eye moves involuntarily, most people think it is a prosthetic eye. Actually, my right eye is the prosthetic one.
> —*Vivian*

If you wear glasses to enhance your remaining vision, you may feel embarrassed by the tint, the thickness of the lenses, or the way they magnify the look of your eyes. Remember that these lenses also magnify your world. By wearing your glasses, bioptics, or telescopic devices, and by learning to use other visual cues, you can safely and efficiently move about in the world.

Traveling Tool

Many people who use a cane for the first time may feel embarrassed or awkward. Since cane users are often depicted on TV or in movies as bumbling, tapping subjects for comedy, you may feel reluctant to cast yourself in this light. But take a moment to really observe an experienced cane user before you decide to write off the cane as a traveling tool. As the person experienced with the cane walks down the street, his movements are fluid, smooth, and sure. His confidence comes from knowing that the cane will help him locate and move around objects and hazards such as manholes, curbs, cracks, and steps.

Your cane can also give you information about activity on the street. A sweep of the cane tells you that it is garbage pick-up day on Main Street because all the cans are out on the street, or that Elm Avenue has a lot of resident toddlers who like to leave their tricycles on the sidewalk during lunch. If you use a cane and have usable residual vision, you may want to use the cane to view objects in your path and use your residual vision to enjoy the scenery around you.

Those who have unusable residual vision or progressive eye conditions may find that learning to use a cane is the most efficient means of travel. This may also be true for people who have night blindness. Good cane traveling skills are always an asset and are a prerequisite for dog guide training.

Dog Guides

If you add a dog guide to the picture, you should be able to move even more quickly and surely. The dog circumnavigates hazards that you would have to first identify with a cane, or constantly check visually, then react to. The public also often reacts more positively to a dog guide. You may find that strangers do not hesitate to talk to you about your dog. A dog guide can be a great ice-breaker.

Do not make the mistake of thinking that your dog guide is in control. That privilege still belongs to you. Since dogs cannot read street maps or identify colors, you must still pay attention to where you are going. You must also depend on auditory clues to tell you when to cross the street. Dog guides require much care, attention, time, love, and discipline. However, if one fits your needs, you may find that your dog guide is both a traveling partner and a great companion.

When you think about it, all of these aids are no more embarrassing than a jeweler's eyepiece, a navigator's compass, or a mountain climber's pitons. They merely help you take advantage of the remaining sight you have and enable you to avoid danger. What is so embarrassing about that?

Of course, we would be less than honest if we did not note that you probably will come across some embarrassing situations while traveling. Let's see if we can give you a new way to look at them.

Crossing Streets

Imagine that you are patiently waiting to cross a street corner and someone grabs your hand and pulls you across the street in order to "help" you. We tend to liken this person to the Boy Scout who will do a good deed for you even if it kills you. We figure that he is the one who should feel embarrassed. After all, he made the mistake, not you. Tell him that you are quite competent and will let him know if you need his assistance.

When you cross the street without assistance, use your usable residual vision and optical aids to locate the "Walk" and "Don't Walk" signs, the crosswalk lines, and the spot where the street islands begin and end. Position yourself so that you can read the bus numbers while you wait at the bus stop. At busy, complex intersections, allow yourself all the time you need and do not allow anyone to hurry you.

> **Journal Note:** Don't be afraid to take as much time as you need with your new optical aids. Sometimes I would wait through three traffic lights to make sure I had seen everything I wanted to see at a complex traffic crossing.
>
> *—Vivian*

What if you veer a little and cross kitty-corner instead of straight across when you attempt to cross the street? If you are using your cane or a dog guide or wearing opticaids, it will be apparent that you have a visual impairment and motorists will probably respond appropriately and courteously. The motorists will have information about you and will not assume that you are just not paying attention. Don't be embarrassed if you make a navigational error.

Even if you are traveling with someone's assistance, you still can end up in a sticky situation. Using the sighted guide technique, many a novice will walk you into a post. When this happens, use humor. Say "What's the matter with you? Are you blind or something?" Humor will defuse a potentially embarrassing situation and let your guide feel more relaxed and, hopefully, better able to guide you because he will be more aware of what to watch for.

Humor Me

Try to handle embarrassing situations with humor. If you mistake a gentleman's lap for an empty seat on the bus, just laugh and say, "Well, that would have been a comfortable seat, but I'll try one of my own!" Use your other senses and tools to help you avoid these embarrassing situations by feeling for an empty seat with your hand, shin, or cane, or by commanding your dog to find one for you. Of course, if your dog directs you to a lap, you can always blame it on him!

Journal Note: Humor has helped me through many an embarrassing situation. One time at a restaurant counter, the waitress handed me my French fries. I was starving so I dug right in only to hear my neighbor's voice saying, "I believe those are MY fries." The situation just struck me funny and I told him that I would pay him back a handful of fries when my order arrived.
—*Vivian*

Enjoy Life, Eat Out Often

Eating and dining out are rife with opportunities for embarrassing situations. To start with, the waitress or waiter may ask your companion what you want to order instead of addressing you directly. You can set the situation straight by saying, "Excuse me, are you speaking to me?" or "I can order for myself." The server may become embarrassed, but that's okay. It is a good learning experience for him.

If you are busy trying to cut your meat and carry on a conversation at the same time, you may not remember that your glass of milk is next to your plate until it has spilled to the floor. To avoid these accidents, try to place your glass out of harm's way. If you are the type of person given to frequent and expansive hand gestures, remove all objects near your plate to a safer spot. When a spill occurs, offer to wipe it up and move on. Everybody does these kinds of things, sighted or not.

In order to avoid playing "Guess the Mystery Meat," ask your waitress or eating companion to describe where each item is on your plate. Ask him to picture your plate as a big clock and to tell you what is at each number, such as carrots at 8 o'clock and salad at 3 o'clock. Although you may be able to easily see the dark meat, the mashed potatoes may be camouflaged against the white dinnerware.

Ask your companion to tell you where everything else is on the table. He should let you know the location of your water glass, the salt and pepper shakers, the centerpiece, and so on. If you are alone, systematically explore the table with your fingers.

If you have been sharing a pizza and want to subtly find out if there is any left (rather than feeling in the box), say something such as, "That pizza was great. Would you mind if I have another piece?" Tell your companions what is on your mind and allow them to give you feedback and information. This will help put them at ease.

Tell your companion that you want to be told if you spill something or if you have some food on your face. When he tells you, take care of it and carry on. If you know that you are going out for barbecued spareribs, you may want to avoid wearing your white shirt and opt for a dark one that will disguise any mishaps.

You Could Have Fooled Me

In time, you may become so adroit at traveling and doing your everyday chores that people will not realize you are visually impaired. This can also lead to embarrassing circumstances. For instance, when you are at the grocery store trying to pick a good green pepper for your favorite pepper stew recipe, you may have difficulty telling the red pepper from the green. When you ask a fellow shopper for help, mention that you are visually impaired so he will know why you are asking. Otherwise, your actions might be misinterpreted.

> **Journal Note:** There are so many embarrassing situations, I don't know which one to choose. While waiting in an airport to go to Portugal, my husband and I decided to relax and sit down in the waiting area. While trying to locate an empty chair (my husband was looking away at this moment), I inadvertently reached for a foreign passenger's crotch. By this time, my husband saw what happened. We showed the couple my white cane and tried to explain that I was blind. Since

this couple didn't speak any English, I hope they did get the message.

—*Rachael*

Journal Note: Many people have commented that they didn't know I was blind until they saw me use my cane to get around.

—*Frank*

Misinterpretation often occurs when your traveling aids are not in plain sight. If you are sitting on the bus or taking a breather from doing laps in the community pool, your eyes may come into contact with someone else's eyes. Unknown to you, you have made eye contact and the other person may think you are staring or trying to open a conversation. When this happens, the other person will often say, "Hi," or something less friendly such as, "What are you staring at?" To the latter you could reply, "Gee, since I have limited vision, I wasn't really staring at anything." To the friendlier opener you could say, "Hi, I'm visually impaired. I hope I didn't appear to be staring at you," and take it from there.

When you say you are visually impaired, do not be disturbed if the other person replies, "Oh, I'm sorry!" He is speaking off the top of his head and seconds later will probably feel embarrassed about his comment. You can help him out by saying, "That's okay, I'm doing fine," or "I'm not sorry, that's just the way it is." If you say it with a smile and a relaxed air, you will both feel at ease.

Mannerisms To Avoid

Unknown to you, you may be developing some mannerisms that are embarrassing to others around you. These may include constantly putting your fingers in or near your eyes, keeping your head down, rocking, excessively touching or adjusting your optical aids, constant, fixated staring, or maintaining a blank, expressionless face.

You need to speak frankly with your loved ones and friends. Ask them to tell you if you exhibit any of these mannerisms. Explain that since you want to know when your slip is showing or when you have spaghetti sauce on your lip, you also want to know if you are developing blind mannerisms. Take a few moments to explain to your loved ones what you can and cannot see and how you must hold your head to see best. Since people gather many clues from their companion's face during a conversation, it is important to look as if you are listening. This came naturally when you were sighted. Now that you are losing your sight, you may be concentrating so hard on what your companion is saying or doing or on the environment around you, that your face is not free to react. You may have to practice "active" listening.

Choose a time when you are alone, and look at or listen to a television or radio program. As the person talks or reads new items, allow your face to mirror the emotional reactions you feel. This may feel strange at first, but you may improve communication with those around you by learning to listen with an animated face.

> **Journal Note:** When working on my own facial expressions, it was quite a challenge to learn the difference between a wink and a blink. It was hard for my sighted friends to tell me the difference and to practice.
> —*Vivian*

As a friend or relative, use tact when you point out these mannerisms. Be direct, but matter-of-fact. Try something such as, "Dad, I know you are concentrating on what I'm saying or what you're seeing, but when you look down, I don't get any eye contact with you. Do you think you could look in the direction of my voice?"

The same holds true for telling your loved one about a

stained suit or uncombed hair. Let them know (in private) about the potentially embarrassing situation and then move on to other things. Just think about how you would want to be treated and you will probably do fine.

Organizational Checklist

- Investigate tinted or dark glasses if you are uncomfortable with the appearance of your eyes.
- Use all your aids, including travel aids, openly.
- Ask about the location of things in a room, on the table, or on a plate.
- Be aware of distracting mannerisms.
- Look in the direction of the speaker.
- Practice facial expressions.
- Look for the humor in embarrassing situations.
- Ask friends and relatives to announce when they enter or leave a room, especially when you are in an unfamiliar environment.

12

The Rehabilitation Program

Remember your first day of school? You probably felt anxious and apprehensive. You may have wondered, "What will the teacher think of me?" "What will happen if I can't do everything I am supposed to do?" "Will my family be happy with what I learn?" and "How will I learn everything?" You may experience those same feelings again when you consider entering a formal rehabilitation program. It may seem easier to just go on as you have been, learning your own ways and adapting tasks using a trial-and-error approach.

When you think about it, the trial-and-error approach has a lot of drawbacks. It usually takes longer and the errors have a way of becoming more of a trial than you thought they would be.

> **Journal Note:** Prior to rehabilitation training, I did not want anyone to know that I had a vision impairment. Now that I have been provided with adaptive skills, I feel that I can go anywhere in the world without getting lost. I feel that life is full of trial and error. If you don't use your capabilities, they will deteriorate.
>
> —*Rose*

You may want to participate in a formal rehabilitation program. Rehabilitation teachers and counselors have been trained to provide you with safe, alternative techniques and adaptive skills that will allow you to perform the necessary activities of daily living. They will also assist you in setting reasonable goals.

You will not be pressured to learn anything you do not want to learn, so don't look at formal rehabilitation as an "all or nothing" exercise. After all, you are not storming the beach at Normandy, you are just taking a series of steps on the road to independence. When you feel you are ready to participate in formal rehabilitation training, look up the phone number for the **State Department of Rehabilitation**, or the **Commission for the Blind**, or **Services for the Blind** in the telephone book and call them.

The name of the state agency that handles rehabilitation services and the curriculum and training of rehabilitation programs may vary from state to state. These state agencies may provide a variety of services, such as counseling, training, referrals, job site evaluations, and so on. This chapter describes the formal rehabilitation program offered in California, because it features many facets of any comprehensive state rehabilitation program.

Teacher/Counselor

Once you make contact, you will be assigned a teacher/counselor for the blind who probably will make an appointment to visit you (and your family, if you want) at home or on the job. During your initial consultation, the teacher/counselor will work with you to assess and determine realistic goals.

Be prepared to answer a lot of questions. Your counselor will need to have information about your general medical status and physical limitations, visual fields and acuity, visual functional limitations, education, employment history, and financial status. She will also take into consideration factors such as your age, social and recreational needs, motivational level, psychological readiness, personal support system (friends and family), professional support system (clergy and personal counselor), and your knowledge of community resources that will meet your visual impairment and personal needs.

During your initial interview, remember that your teacher/counselor is not being nosy. She needs to draw a clear profile of you in order to help you set up a course of training that will allow you to achieve the goals appropriate for you.

During your interview, she may ask you to have a hearing test to determine your current level of hearing. You are required by the California State Department of Rehabilitation to produce documentation of the status of your physical health, visual impairment, hearing level, and any functional limitations you may have. Your doctor can provide these to you or to the Department on request.

The California State Department of Rehabilitation also needs to have documentation that shows if there is reasonable expectation that you will benefit from rehabilitation services. In other words, the Department needs to feel that you would be a willing participant in the rehabilitation process and that you are physically able to use the skills they will teach you. Rehabilitation counseling and training are usually provided free in California. The teacher/counselor for the visually impaired will talk with you about how you are coping with personal management (grooming and eating skills), household management (cooking and household tasks), money management (system for identifying and organizing money), communication management (reading and writing braille, typing, handwriting), and orientation and mobility skills (traveling).

For those of you who are planning to return to work, your teacher/counselor will assess your prevocational skills (braille, typing skills, using public transit, and so on). With your permission, she will share this information with a vocational rehabilitation counselor for the blind. This counselor will handle the evaluation and goal-setting process related to employment.

Perhaps you are already retired or are permanently unable to return to work and want to learn how to prepare meals, clean your home, and maintain your yard using your limited vision.

Perhaps you can still do your job but want to learn how to use the public transit system. Will your counselor for the visually impaired allow you to learn what YOU want to learn? Yes, your teacher/counselor will work with you to evaluate your skills and assist you in developing realistic goals that you want to achieve.

However, this is a team effort and you have to do your part. Do not be a passive bystander during your initial interview, especially if family members are present and want to do the talking for you. You must be firm about stating the goals you want to achieve—apart from those your family or counselor may want you to achieve. Ask questions about things that are unclear. Ask for information about groups and organizations for the visually impaired. These groups may meet for social, recreational, or discussion purposes.

Plan of Action

Your teacher/counselor for the blind will then write a formal report, or Individualized Written Rehabilitation Plan (IWRP). You will be given a copy of this report. It will list the goals you want to reach, methods for achieving these goals, and a reasonable time line in which to accomplish your rehabilitation objectives. A sample IWRP might read like this:

Individualized Written Rehabilitation Plan
Mrs. Jones is visually impaired as a result of age-related maculopathy. As a result of this client's visual impairment, she is unable to:

- Prepare meals safely.
- Travel independently.
- Perform sewing tasks.
- Read standard print.

- Perform household and personal management tasks.
- Write (correspond with the sighted world).

In order that Mrs. Jones obtain the necessary adaptive skills to perform activities of daily living, the following services are recommended:

1. Braille instructions will enable this client to keep track of phone numbers and notes.

2. Typing lessons will provide a means for communicating with the sighted world. A signature guide will enable this client to sign correspondence.

3. Sewing and cooking tips will provide adaptive ways to perform these activities. Adaptive aids, such as a magnifier for machine sewing and machine markings, are recommended.

   To enhance previously learned skills, during cooking lessons, this client will be introduced to cooking and safety tips and adaptive cooking devices—such as a liquid level indicator, vegetable/tomato slicer, and elbow-length oven mitts.

4. Mobility training will enable Mrs. Jones to go independently to her doctor appointments and senior citizen functions.

   During orientation and mobility instruction, she will learn to use her usable residual vision, along with a rigid long white cane, in order to ride public transportation independently.

5. Tips about how to conduct activities of daily living will enable this client to use alternative techniques to perform light housekeeping duties and personal management tasks.

6. Adjustment to blindness counseling will provide an opportunity for Mrs. Jones to express her feelings, fears, and concerns regarding her visual impairment.

7. Adaptive home aids, such as a talking calculator, braille watch, large print label maker, and a page magnifier, will enable this client to further her independence in her home. Procurement of Hi-Marks labeling paste will enable Mrs. Jones to mark appliances at appropriate settings.

As a result of rehabilitation services, Mrs. Jones will be able to resume functioning independently in her own home and in her community. She will no longer be dependent on family members and/or governmental homemaker services for support.

Resources

As a part of the rehabilitation process, your teacher/counselor for the visually impaired will inform you about your rights to federal and state disability, unemployment, and welfare benefits, and may possibly be available to help you in completing the paper work if necessary. She will tell you about available community resources and give you the names and phone numbers of organizations that can further inform you about your visual impairment needs.

> **Journal Note:** My wife and I receive Supplemental Social Security Income. My wife is a full-time homemaker and mother. Although I have a B.A. in physical education, I have been unable to obtain full-time employment. Through adult education, I presently teach exercise classes for the visually impaired at a nearby center for the blind. In addition to this, I volunteer to help out in a ceramics class at the center.
>
> —*John*

New Places, New Faces

You may learn your adaptive techniques of daily living in one of a variety of settings. You may learn in your own home, in an independent living center (an apartment setting), in a state-regulated dormitory setting, or in a local community center for the blind. As a general rule, in California the independent living center tends to be used by congenitally blind people who are emerging adults and have never lived independently, whereas the state-regulated dormitory setting is geared toward adults who are newly blind.

Those who learn in an independent living center, or apartment setting, live in an apartment and learn to set up house, cook, iron, clean, manage money, pay bills, touch-type, learn braille, and use orientation and mobility skills on these premises and in the community.

Those who learn in a state-regulated dormitory setting live in the dorms and go to classrooms to learn independent living skills, personal management, orientation and mobility, touch-typing, braille instruction, household management, money management, and shop skills such as woodworking. This type of setting is for adults who are newly blind and prefer to learn all the adaptive skills simultaneously.

> **Journal Note:** Given that I was sighted one day and totally blind the next, I am very glad that I was immediately provided with rehabilitation services in order to cope and live with my blindness. During the first four months of being newly blind, I was provided with orientation and mobility training, cooking instructions, organizational tips, and braille lessons in my home. Since I wanted to regain my independence as soon as possible, I was referred by my rehabilitation counselor to the Orientation Center for the Blind in Albany, California. This training environment enabled me to see how other newly blind people function and to learn how to deal with fears related to blindness.
>
> —*Janice*

Those who learn in a local community center for the blind often live at home and go to the center for instruction. These services vary from offering fully accredited, formal rehabilitation programs to providing only social and recreational activities.

You may also learn skills by correspondence course. The Hadley School for the Blind in Winnetka, Illinois, offers taped courses that cover such subjects as braille instruction, child care, computer operation, foreign languages, high school diploma, touch-typing, medical transcription, and so on.

> **Journal Note:** I am glad I was provided with rehabilitation services for the blind. Services were provided to me in and out of my home. During the beginning of my training, I was provided with organizational tips and traveling instructions, and was introduced to adaptive aids. I attended the Orientation Center for the Blind in Albany, California, for seven months. Those who are partially sighted were taught under blindfold. I feel that this is a good idea because whether your vision fluctuates or not, you know in the back of your mind that you can handle just about any situation.
>
> *—Rose*

Get to Work

If your rehabilitation report includes vocational goals, you will be assigned a vocational rehabilitation counselor for the blind. She will repeat the application and rehabilitation assessment process, stressing your job-related skills.

During the initial interview, your vocational rehabilitation counselor for the blind will need your input to write a report that reflects your personal and vocational needs. As a part of this vocational rehabilitation program report, you may be requested to participate in a vocational evaluation. The evaluation may note your education and academic ability, attitude toward blindness, and motivational and functional limitations in possible job settings. It will also include recommendations for suitable vocational options. The final report will describe the skills you need to learn to do a specific job. It will also describe any retraining you may need, as well as new job possibilities, if necessary. It will list any aids or special equipment you will need to perform a job independently, and include a time line for achieving your vocational rehabilitation objectives.

> **Journal Note:** When I realized that I wouldn't be able to do the type of work I had trained all my life to do, I felt very concerned about how I would continue to be the breadwinner in the family. Thank goodness my employer was able to retrain me and be supportive of my job-related needs.
>
> —*Susan*

In California, you can work on both your prevocational and vocational rehabilitation programs at the same time. You and your two counselors will regularly meet to discuss your rehabilitation/training progress.

Your vocational rehabilitation counselor for the blind may want to conduct a job-site analysis to see which parts of your job you can still do and to determine what is needed to perform all aspects of your job independently. She may be able to advise you about setting up new work systems, such as a new way to file so you can retrieve information quickly and independently. Until you can use adaptive means to perform your job-related tasks, she may suggest ways you can share those parts of the job that are currently inaccessible to you.

> **Journal Note:** I work as a cashier for a fast-food restaurant. I use a braille overlay to identify the cash register keys. I use a voice box that tells me how much people are paying for an order and how much change

I give them back. I use a money teller machine to identify paper money.

—*Emily*

For instance, if you are a classroom elementary school
teacher, your counselor may provide tips for how you can
develop listening skills, as well as alternatives to lesson preparation and presentation.

> **Journal Note:** Besides being a homemaker, I run a
> Christian preschool day-care out of my home. I have a
> teacher and one assistant. When I first meet with par-
> ents, I try to make them feel at ease and let them know
> that their children will have the best care. In getting
> acquainted with a child, I explain to them that my eyes
> are broken and that they are here to help me. There
> are about ten children in my day-care at this time.
>
> —*Rachael*

That makes sense for a teacher, but what if you are a bus
driver? How can a vocational counselor help you? Obviously she
cannot return you to your present job, but she might arrange to
retrain you to become a bus dispatcher. Since you already know
the routes, you would be a natural. Or perhaps you decide
together that you would be better suited to customer service,
helping the public plan their routes to work or school. She would
introduce you to braille or large print maps and teach you braille
and communication and phone skills.

> **Journal Note:** When it was determined that I would
> no longer be able to do my job due to safety reasons,
> I went on disability leave. I received compensation for
> the same amount of regular pay. During my disability
> leave, I participated in a rehabilitation program for
> the visually impaired. I learned how to read and write
> braille, how to use a long white cane for traveling,
> and adjustment counseling to blindness was provided

for me and my family. I am glad that I had a blind rehabilitation counselor because he was able to communicate what I was going through to my family. My rehab counselor worked with my company to determine what type of job would be suitable for my needs. My employer paid for a low vision examination to determine if visual aids would be helpful for me. With the help of my rehab counselor and company personnel, I was able to continue my employment with this company.

—Susan

What if you want to become a cabinetmaker and the counselor does not know knotty pine from balsa wood? Your vocational counselor will assist you in finding training appropriate to your needs and the job market. This may include on-the-job training, an apprenticeship, or enrollment in college courses. Volunteer work in a prospective job may also help you decide if a particular vocation is right for you. Or you can investigate and attend job fairs for the disabled to meet prospective employers and fellow blind job-seekers.

Journal Note: My dad was a candy maker for many years and one of his specialties was caramel corn. He worked with the Department of Rehabilitation to train a visually impaired man to make caramel corn. The man got a job at a candy store and did very well. His was the second best caramel corn I ever tasted.

—Jill

For the most part, blind and visually impaired employees perform the same types of jobs as their sighted counterparts. The following are just a sampling of occupation possibilities:

actor, administrative assistant, accountant, artist

bus dispatcher, botanist, butcher

cashier, counselor, computer programmer, car mechanic

day-care worker, doctor, dishwasher

electrician, engineer, economist

foreman, fisherman, farmer

gardener, golfer, gas station attendant

health-care worker, hairdresser, housekeeper

industrial consultant, illustrator, insurance salesman

janitor, job analyst, jeweler, judge

key maker, kitchen worker

lawyer, laborer, librarian

medical technician, manager

nutritionist, newspaper reporter

operator, office worker, optician

parent, public servant, producer

quality control worker

realtor, radio announcer, researcher, rehabilitation
    instructor

scientist, secretary, seamstress

teacher, travel agent, translator

union leader, usher

vendor, volunteer worker

waitress/waiter, window washer, woodworker

X-ray technician

zookeeper

The Department of Labor, in partnership with the National
Federation of the Blind, conducts a nationwide program called
Job Opportunities for the Blind (JOB), a program that matches
qualified blind workers with employers. You can contact them at:

Job Opportunities for the Blind
1800 Johnson Street
Baltimore, MD 21230
(410) 659-9314.

Ask for information about the program and descriptions of blind employees in a variety of vocations.

The President's Committee on Employment of People with Disabilities has established an international information clearinghouse and consulting service on practical methods of job accommodations called the Job Accommodation Network (JAN). JAN counsels individuals with disabilities, employers, and rehabilitation professionals seeking job accommodation solutions. The service is free of charge, but JAN does request follow-up information about the success of the accommodation for their computer files. Contact them at:

Job Accommodation Network
West Virginia University
809 Allen Hall, P.O. Box 6123,
Morgantown, WV 26506-6123
(800) JAN-PCEH (526-7234).

The cost of vocational training is usually little or nothing. For those who cannot afford to purchase equipment, clothing for work or school, school tuition, or transportation to school or work (short-term), the California Department of Vocational Rehabilitation will finance them or find the resources, such as grants or loans, that will enable you to finance your rehabilitation needs. The Department determines financial need and training on an individualized basis.

Journal Note: I obtained small engine mechanic training through the State Department of Vocational Rehabilitation. Two months after completing my training, I was able to find employment. I worked nine years for three employers. After being laid off from my third job, I decided to go into business for myself. I have been self-employed for four years and am having success in my business.

—Louis

If it appears that you need or would benefit from psychological counseling regarding adjustment to your visual impairment and this coverage is not offered by your health insurance, the California Rehabilitation Department may provide limited psychological counseling or refer you to public health services that will provide psychological counseling at no cost or on a sliding scale fee basis.

After you have completed your vocational training program, your vocational rehabilitation counselor will provide job-seeking skills, such as resume writing and interviewing tips, to enable you to obtain employment. She may also refer you to job-search and support organizations for the disabled. Some of these may be outside the State Department of Vocational Rehabilitation.

> **Journal Note:** When going for an interview for my third job, the person I interviewed with was very concerned that I might get hurt. I tried to assure him that I had worked with others and that I did not have a problem. About a week later, I went back to the same company and spoke to another fellow who was subordinate to the first man. My second interviewer was so excited about my working there he convinced his boss that the business should give me a chance to prove myself and I was hired.
>
> *—Louis*

A Working Relationship

By now, it may be obvious to you that you are going to be spending a lot of time with your counselor. What does this mean? What should you expect of this counselor?

View her as a concerned counselor and teacher. She will teach you skills, help you become aware of available resources, serve as your advocate, and provide supportive counseling and guidance services.

A teacher/counselor or vocational counselor working in California holds a college degree in a social work (or rehabilitation) related field and has had training and experience working with disabled persons. He or she has completed a year of training covering social and medical issues, situation assessment, goal setting, interviewing techniques, analysis of psychological tests and medical reports, and methods for teaching adaptive techniques of daily living for the visually impaired. Your counselor may or may not be visually impaired.

> **Journal Note:** When I first found out that I was legally blind, I was very frightened. I was constantly worried that I was going to become totally blind. After learning how Vivian, my rehab counselor, functioned and got about with less vision than I had, I felt less afraid and encouraged that I could continue living independently.
> —Gwen

Although your counselor may be friendly, this is really a professional relationship, not a personal friendship. She is not someone you should call in the middle of the night to ask about the meaning of a strange dream. In any case, you probably will not have her home phone number and should not request it. You should not expect her to casually stop by your house or visit you in the hospital. View her as you would a doctor, lawyer, teacher, or any other professional person.

Unfortunately, your counselor is not magic. She will not be able to make everything right for you with a wave of her hand. She may not even know the answers to all of your questions or have the time and resources to inform you of everything. Therefore, she may refer you to other resources so you can discover information on your own. Be willing to accept this part of the partnership.

Your counselor will not expect you to perform perfectly. She just wants you to do your best to accomplish your goals. After all, that is also her goal. Your rehabilitation counselor should be non-judgmental and supportive during both your good days and your bad days. If you have a personality clash with your counselor, explain your concerns to her. If it remains a problem, ask to be reassigned.

Family Connection

As a family member or friend of someone going through a formal or informal rehabilitation program, you can help by being nonjudgmental, patient, and supportive. Do not impose your values or goals on your loved one. You need to be flexible about the time it takes to for get things done, and encouraging if a goal is not reached by a projected date. After all, what difference does it make if he learns braille in six months or seven months? The important thing is that he learn to read braille, right?

If you are a friend or relative of a visually impaired person, let the counselor know that you want to have some training, too. Ask for instruction on how to orient the visually impaired person to his plate. Request that she show you the sighted guide technique (see Chapter 6) for traveling, and ask for tips on how to handle embarrassing or uncomfortable situations you may have encountered. Invite her to tell you how you can encourage your loved one and help him progress in his rehabilitation program.

Encourage family discussions to air concerns. Maybe you are upset that since your visually impaired husband has learned to take the bus to work he must now leave the house earlier and cannot walk the kids to school. Talk about it. Maybe he can compensate by making their lunches the night before, saving you some time in the morning. Try to keep these meetings low-key and solution-oriented.

As your loved one goes through this rehabilitation program, try to resist being overprotective. Do not put limitations on him.

Journal Note: As I watched my husband lose his vision, I became increasingly protective for his safety, especially at work. Often there's construction going on in various parts of the plant.

—Linda

During counseling meetings, let your loved one set his own goals. Comments such as, "But, Dad, you shouldn't learn to cook, you'll burn the house down," "You shouldn't learn to travel outside the house, you'll fall!" or "You can't be retrained, you're too set in your ways," are discouraging, defeatist, and probably farfetched. Let him know that you love him, have faith in him, and that you know he can do the job, one way or another.

Organizational Checklist

- Call the Department of Rehabilitation and make an appointment with a rehabilitation counselor.
- Ask your doctor for documentation of visual impairment.
- Make a list of tasks or rehabilitation goals you want to get done.
- Investigate correspondence courses.
- Contact Job Opportunities for the Blind or Job Accommodation Network if necessary.
- Refer to *The Post-Secondary Education and Career Development: A Resource Guide for the Blind and Visually Impaired and Physically Handicapped*, available through the National Federation of the Blind, for examples of employment opportunities.

Appendix

Appendices

Appendix A
Adaptive Aids Catalogs

American Foundation for the Blind
Products for People with Vision Problems
15 West 16th Street
New York, NY 10011

American Printing House for the Blind, Inc.
1839 Frankfort Ave.
P.O. Box 6085
Louisville, KY 40206

BIT Corporation
52 Roland Street
Boston, MA 02129
(1-800) 333-2481 or (800) 333-BIT-1
or FAX (617) 666-4646

Independent Living Aids
27 East Mall
Plainview, NY 11803-4404
(800) 537-2118

LS&S Group, Inc.
P.O. Box 673
Northbrook, IL 60065
(708) 498-9777 or (800) 468-4789

National Association for Visually Handicapped
22 West 21st Street
New York, NY 10010
(212) 889-3141

Appendix B
Companies

American Thermoform Corporation
2311 Travers Avenue
City of Commerce, CA 90040
(213) 723-9021 or FAX (213) 728-8877

Arkenstone, Inc.
1185 Bordeaux Dr. #D
Sunnyvale, CA 94089-1210
(408) 752-2200

Artic Technologies
55 Park Street
Troy, MI 48083-2753
(313) 588-7370 or FAX (313) 588-2650

Berkeley Systems, Inc.
1700 Shattuck Avenue
Berkeley, CA 94709
(415) 540-5535

Blazie Engineering
3660 Mill Green Road
Street, MD 21154
(301) 879-4944 or FAX (301) 452-5752

Boswell Industries, Inc.
Suite 360, 470 Granville Street
Vancouver, BC V6C 1V5, Canada
(604) 684-3629

Computerized Books for the Blind
and Print Handicapped
University of Montana
33 N. Corbin Hall
Missoula, MT 59812
(406) 243-5481

Enabling Technologies Company
3102 S.E. Jay Street
Stuart, FL 34997
(407) 283-4817

Henter-Joyce, Inc.
10901-C Roosevelt Blvd. Suite 1200
St. Petersburg, FL 33716
(813) 576-5658 or FAX (813) 579-4597

HumanWare, Inc.
6245 King Road
Loomis, CA 95650
(916) 652-7253 or FAX (916) 652-7296

IBM National Support Center for Persons
with Disabilities
P.O. Box 2150
Atlanta, GA 30055
(800) 426-2133 (voice) or (800) 284-9482 (TDD)

Lyon Computer Discourse Limited
1009 Kinloch Lane
North Vancouver, BC V7G 1V8, Canada
(604) 929-8886 or FAX (604) 929-8858

Noir Medical Technologies
P.O. Box 159
South Lyon, MI 48178
(313) 769-5565 or (800) 521-9746

Opteq Vision Systems
17355 Mierow Lane
Brookfield, WI 53005
(414) 784-4979

Raised Dot Computing
408 S. Baldwin Street
Madison, WI 53703
(608) 257-9595

Seeing Eye Technologies, Inc.
7074 Brooklyn Boulevard
Minneapolis, MN 55429
(612) 560-8080 or (800) 462-3738
or FAX (612) 560-0663

Talking Computers, Inc.
140 Little Falls Road
Falls Church, VA 22046
(703) 241-8224 or (800) 458-6338

Telesensory Systems, Inc.
455 North Bernardo Avenue
P.O. Box 7455
Mountain View, CA 94039-7455
(415) 960-0920 or (800) 227-8418

Transceptor Technologies, Inc.
P.O. Box 15771
Ann Arbor, MI 48106-5771
(313) 996-1899

Appendix C
Disability Databases

ABLEDATA
4407 8th Street, N.E.
Washington, DC 20017
800-344-5405

Accent on Information
P.O. Box 700
Bloomington, IL 61701

Ageline
The American Association of Retired Persons
1909 K Street, N.W.
Washington, DC 20049
(202) 872-4700

Assistive Device Database System
Assistive Device Resource Center
California State University
6000 J Street
Sacramento, CA 95819
(916) 454-6422

BCN: Business Computer Network
1046 Central Parkway South
San Antonio, TX 78232
(800) 446-6255

BRS Information Technologies
1200 Route 7
Latham, NY 12110
(800) 345-4BRS

CHID (Combined Health Information Database)
2115 East Jefferson, Suite 401
Rockville, MD 20852
(301) 468-2162

CompuServe
P.O. Box 20212
5000 Arlington Center Boulevard
Columbus, OH 43220
(800) 848-8199

CTG (Closing the Gap) Solutions
P.O. Box 68
Henderson, MN 56044
(612) 248-3294

Dialog Information Services
3460 Hillview Avenue
Palo Alto, CA 94304
(800) 227-1927 or (415) 858-3785

DIG - EL PASO
12907 18th Avenue, South
Burnsville, MN 55337
(612) 894-2991

EASYNET
134 North Narberth Avenue
Narberth, PA
(215) 664-6972

Job Accommodation Network (JAN)
West Virginia University
809 Allen Hall, P.O. Box 6123
Morgantown, WV 26506-6123
800-JAN-PCEH (TTY/TDD)

LOGO
The Young People's Logo Association (YPLA)
P.O. Box 855067
Richardson, TX 75801
(214) 783-7548

Medline
National Library of Medicine
MEDLARS Management Section
8600 Rockville Pike
Bethesda, MD 29209
(301) 496-6193

REHABDATA
The National Rehabilitation Information Center (NARIC)
8455 Colesville Road, Suite 935
Silver Spring, Maryland 20910-3319
(800) 34-NARIC or (301) 588-9284

SPECIALNET
Directors of Special Education
Suite 315, 2021 K Street, N.W.
Washington, DC 20006
(202) 296-1800

TECHNET
The Resource Center for the Handicapped
20150 45th Avenue, N.E.
Seattle, WA 98155
(206) 362-2273

Appendix D
Dog Guide Schools

Eye Dog Foundation for the Blind, Inc.
512 N. Larchmont Boulevard
Los Angeles, CA 90004
(213) 626-3370 or (213) 468-8856

Eye of the Pacific Guide Dogs and Mobility Services, Inc.
747 Amana Street, #407
Honolulu, HI 96814
(808) 941-1088

Fidelco Guide Dog Foundation, Inc.
P.O. Box 142
Bloomfield, CT 06002
(203) 243-5200

Guide Dog Foundation for the Blind, Inc.
371 East Jericho Turnpike
Smithtown, NY 11787
(516) 265-2121

Guide Dogs for the Blind, Inc.
P.O. Box 1200
San Rafael, CA 94915
(415) 479-4000

Guiding Eyes for the Blind, Inc.
611 Granite Springs Road
Yorktown Heights, NY 10598
(914) 245-4024

International Guiding Eyes, Inc.
13445 Glenoaks Boulevard
Sylmar, CA 91342
(213) 362-5834

Leader Dogs for the Blind
1039 Rochester Road
Rochester, MI 48063
(313) 651-9011

Pilot Dogs, Inc.
625 West Town Street
Columbus, OH 43215
(614) 221-6367

Seeing Eye, Inc.
P.O. Box 375
Morristown, NJ 07960
(201) 539-4425

Southeast Guide Dogs, Inc.
4210 77th Street East
Palmetto, FL 33561
(813) 729-5665

Appendix E
Federal Agencies

U.S. Department of Education

Clearinghouse on the Handicapped
330 C Street, S.W., Room 3132
Washington, DC 20202
(202) 732-1241

Division of Blind and Visually Impaired
330 C Street, S.W.
Washington, DC 20202
(202) 732-1316

National Council on the Handicapped
330 C Street, S.W., Room 3118
Washington, DC 20202
(202) 453-3846

National Institute on Disability and Rehabilitation Research
330 C Street, S.W.
Washington, DC 20202
(202) 732-1139

Office of Special Education and Rehabilitative Services
330 C Street, S.W., Room 3132
Washington, DC 20202
(202) 732-1241

Office of Special Education Programs
330 C Street, S.W., Room 3086
Washington, DC 20202
(202) 732-1007

Rehabilitative Services Administration
330 C Street, S.W.
Washington, DC 20202
(202) 732-1282

U.S. Department of Health and Human Services

Administration on Aging
North Building, Room 4760
200 Independence Avenue, S.W.
Washington, DC 20201
(202) 245-0724

Health Resources and Services Administration
Bureau of Health Professions
5600 Fishers Lane
Rockville, MD 20857
(301) 443-5794

National Institutes of Health/National Eye Institute
Building 31, Room AO3
Bethesda, MD 20892
(301) 496-2234

Social Security Administration
6401 Security Boulevard
Baltimore, MD 21235
(301) 965-1234

U.S. Department of Labor

Employment Standards Administration
Branch of Special Employment
200 Constitution Avenue, N.W.
Washington, DC 20210
(202) 523-8727

Office of Federal Contract Compliance Programs
200 Constitution Avenue, N.W.
Washington, DC 20210
(202) 523-9475

U.S. Employment Service
Patrick Henry Building
601 D Street, N.W.
Washington, DC 20213
(202) 376-6750

Veterans Administration

Blind Rehabilitation Service
810 Vermont Avenue, N.W.
Washington, DC 20420

(202) 233-3232
Department of Veterans Benefits
810 Vermont Avenue, N.W.
Washington, DC 20420
(202) 233-2044

Other Agencies

Equal Employment Opportunity Commission
Office of Legal Counsel
2401 E Street, N.W., Room 222
Washington, DC 20507
(202) 634-6460

Library of Congress National Library Service for the Blind and
Physically
Handicapped
1291 Taylor Street, N.W.
Washington, DC 20542
(202) 287-5100 or (1-800) 424-9100

President's Committee on Employment of People with
Disabilities
1331 F Street, N.W., Suite 300
Washington, DC 20004
(202) 653-5044

Small Business Administration
1441 L Street, N.W.
Washington, DC 20416
(202) 653-6605

U.S. Department of Justice
Civil Rights Division/Coordination and Review Section
10th Street and Constitution Avenue, N.W.
Washington, DC 20530
(202) 633-2151 or TDD (telecommunication device for the
deaf) (202) 724-7678

Appendix F
National Organizations

American Association of the Deaf-Blind
814 Thayer Avenue
Silver Spring, MD 20910

American Council of the Blind, Inc.
1155 15th St. N.W. Suite 720
Washington, DC 20005
(202) 467-5081

American Council of the Blind Parents
c/o American Council of the Blind
1010 Vermont Avenue, N.W., Suite 1100
Washington, DC 20005
(202) 393-3666

American Diabetes Association
National Service Center
P.O. Box 25757
1600 Duke Street
Alexandria, VA 22313
(703) 549-1500

American Foundation for the Blind
15 West 16th Street
New York, NY 10011
(212) 620-2000 or (800) 232-5463

Association for Education and Rehabilitation
of the Blind and Visually Impaired
206 North Washington Street, Suite 320
Alexandria, VA 22314
(703) 548-1884

Association for Macular Diseases
210 East 64th Street
New York, NY 10021
(212) 605-3719

Association for Persons with Severe Handicaps, The (TASH)
7010 Roosevelt Way, N.E.
Seattle, WA 98115
(206) 523-8446

Association of Radio Reading Services
P.O. Box 847
Lawrence, KS 66044
(913) 864-4600

Association on Handicapped Student Service Programs
        in Postsecondary Education
P.O. Box 21192
Columbus, OH 43221
(614) 488-4872

Blind Outdoor Leisure Development
533 East Main Street
Aspen, CO 81611
(303) 925-8922

Blinded Veterans Association
1726 M Street, N.W., Suite 800
Washington, DC 20036
(202) 223-3066

Council for Exceptional Children
1920 Association Drive
Reston, VA 22091
(703) 620-3660

Council of Citizens with Low Vision International
5707 Brockton Drive, #302
Indianapolis, IN 46220-5481
(616) 381-9566

Council of Rehabilitation Specialists
c/o American Council of the Blind
1010 Vermont Avenue, N.W., Suite 1100
Washington, DC 20005
(202) 376-0442

Foundation for Glaucoma Research
490 Post Street, Suite 1042
San Francisco, CA 94102
(415) 986-3162

Guide Dog Users
2130 Maple Street
Baldwin, NY 11510
(312) 848-6191

Helen Keller International
15 West 16th Street
New York, NY 10011
(212) 807-5800

Helen Keller National Center for Deaf-Blind Youths and Adults
111 Middle Neck Road
Sands Point, NY 11050
(516) 944-8900 (voice and TDD)

Job Accommodation Network (JAN)
West Virginia University
809 Allen Hall, P.O. Box 6123
Morgantown, WV 26506-6123
(800) JAN-PCEH (526-7234)

Job Opportunities for the Blind
National Federation of the Blind
1800 Johnson Street
Baltimore, MD 21230
(301) 659-9314

Lions Club International
300 22nd Street
Oak Brook, IL 60570
(312) 571-5466

Myasthenia Gravis Foundation
7-11 South Broadway
White Plains, NY 10601
(914) 328-1717

National Association for Parents of the Visually Impaired, Inc.
P.O. Box 317
Watertown, MA 02272
(800) 562-6265

National Association for Visually Handicapped
22 West 21st Street
New York, NY 10010
(212) 889-3141

National Braille Association
1290 University Avenue
Rochester, NY 14607
(716) 473-0900

National Eye Institute
Bldg. 31, Room AO3
Bethesda, MD 20892
(301) 496-2234

National Eye Research Foundation
910 Skokie Blvd.
Northbrook, IL 60062
(312) 564-4652

National Federation of the Blind
1800 Johnson Street
Baltimore, MD 21230
(410) 659-9314

National Industries for the Blind
524 Hamburg Turnpike
Wayne, NJ 07470
(201) 595-9200

National Multiple Sclerosis Society
733 Third Avenue
New York, NY 10017
(212) 986-3240

National Society to Prevent Blindness
500 East Remington Road
Schaumburg, IL 60173
(312) 843-2020

National Rehabilitation Information Center
Suite 935
8455 Colesville Road
Silver Spring, MD 20910-3319
(301) 588-9284

President's Committee on Employment of People with
Disabilities
Suite 300
1331 F Street, N.W.
Washington, D.C. 20004
(202) 653-5044

Randolph-Sheppard Vendors of America
c/o Paul Verner
7505 Robindale Road
Tampa, FL 33619
(813) 272-2300

Recording for the Blind
20 Roszel Road
Princeton, NJ 08540
(609) 452-0606

RP Foundation Fighting Blindness (National Retinitis
Pigmentosa Foundation, Inc.)
1401 Mt. Royal Avenue, Fourth Floor
Baltimore, MD 21217

Sensory Aids Foundation
Suite 12
399 Sherman Avenue
Palo Alto, CA 94306
(415) 329-0430

Smith-Kettlewell Eye Research Institute
2232 Webster Street
San Francisco, CA 94115
(415) 561-1619

Telephone Pioneers of America
22 Cortlandt Street
Room C-2575
New York, NY 10007
(212) 393-3252

Tel-Med
952 South Mt. Vernon Avenue
Colton, CA 92324
(714) 825-6034

United States Association for Blind Athletes
33 N. Institute Street
Brown Hall, Suite 015
Colorado Springs, CO 80903
(719) 630-0422

Appendix G
Periodicals

ACB Parents Newsletter
Council of Citizens with Low Vision
Education Office
Tower 2, #2102
600 N. Alabama Street
Indianapolis, IN 46204-1415

AER Report
Association for Education and Rehabilitation
of the Blind and Visually Impaired
206 N. Washington Street, #320
Alexandria, VA 22314
(703) 548-1884

AFB News
American Foundation for the Blind
15 West 16th Street
New York, NY 10011
(212) 620-2000

The American Lupus Society Quarterly
The American Lupus Society
23751 Madison Street
Torrance, CA 90505
(213) 373-1335

Blindskills, Inc.
Box 5181
Salem, OR 97304
503 581-4224

Blindness, Visual Impairment, Deaf-Blindness:
Semiannual Listing of Current Literature
Association for Education of the Visually Handicapped
919 Walnut Street, Room 700
Philadelphia, PA 19107

Braille Book Review
National Library Service for the Blind
and Physically Handicapped
1291 Taylor Street, N.W.
Washington, DC 20542
(202) 287-5000

Braille Forum
American Council of the Blind
1155 15th St. N.W. Suite 720
Washington, DC 20005
(202) 467-5081

Braille Monitor
National Federation of the Blind
1800 Johnson Street
Baltimore, MD 21230
(301) 659-9314

CCLV Newsletter
Council of Citizens with Low Vision
Education Office
Tower 2, #2102
600 N. Alabama Street
Indianapolis, IN 46204-1415
(317) 635-4419

Diabetes '90
American Diabetes Association
1660 Duke Street
Alexandria, VA 22314
(703) 549-1500

Education of the Visually Handicapped
Heldref Publications
4000 Albemarle Street, N.W.
Washington, DC 20016

Encore
Division for the Blind and Physically Handicapped
Library of Congress
Washington, DC 20540

Hearsay
Association of Radio Reading Services
National Office
4200 Wisconsin Avenue, N.W., Suite 106-346
Washington, DC 20016
(202) 347-0955

HKI Report
Helen Keller International
15 W. 16th Street
New York, NY 10011
(212) 807-5860

Inside MS
National Multiple Sclerosis Society
733 Third Avenue
New York, NY 10017-5706
(212) 986-3240

Journal of Visual Impairment and Blindness
American Foundation for the Blind
15 W. 16th Street
New York, NY 10011
(212) 620-2000

Matilda Ziegler Magazine for the Blind
20 W. 17th Street
New York, NY 10011
212 242-0263

NARIC Quarterly
National Rehabilitation Information Center
8455 Colesville Road Suite 935
Silver Spring, MD 20910-3319
(800) 346-2742

NBA Bulletin
National Braille Association
1290 University Avenue
Rochester, NY 14607

NEWSBITS
Talking Computers, Inc.
140 Little Falls Road
Falls Church, VA 22046
(800) 458-6338

Opportunity
National Industries for the Blind
524 Hamburg Turnpike
Wayne, NJ 07470
(201) 595-9200

Recording for the Blind News
20 Roszel Road
Princeton, NJ 08540
(609) 452-0606

Reflections
Council of Citizens with Low Vision
Education Office
Tower 2, #2102
600 N. Alabama Street
Indianapolis, IN 46204-1415
(804) 288-0395

Student Advocate
National Alliance of Blind Students
1010 Vermont Avenue, N.W., Suite 1100
Washington, DC 20005
(202) 393-3666 OR (800) 424-8666

Talking Book Topics
National Library Service for the Blind and Physically
Handicapped
Library of Congress
1291 Taylor Street, N.W.
Washington, DC 20542
(202) 287-5100

Update
National Library Service for the Blind and Physically
Handicapped
Library of Congress
1291 Taylor Street, N.W.
Washington, DC 20542
(202) 287-5100

Vendorscope
Randolph-Sheppard Vendors of America
Council of Citizens with Low Vision
Education Office
Tower 2, #2102
600 N. Alabama Street
Indianapolis, IN 46204-1415

Appendix H
Radio Reading Services

Alabama Radio Reading Service Network
1028 Seventh Avenue South
Birmingham, AL 35294
(205) 934-2606

Arkansas Radio Reading for the Blind, Inc.
P.O. Box 668
Little Rock, AR 72203
(501) 663-4540

Association of Radio Reading Services
c/o Sun Sound Reading Service
3124 East Roosevelt Street
Phoenix, AZ 85008
(800) 255-2777

Baltimore's Radio Reading Service
2901 Liberty Heights Avenue
Baltimore, MD 21215
(301) 396-0990

Broadcast Services for the Blind, Inc.
20 Tenth Street
San Francisco, CA 94103
(415) 431-1481

CenTex
P.O. Box 158
Williamsburg, VA 23185
(804) 229-8541

Central Indiana Radio Reading, Inc.
Butler University, Box 110
Indianapolis, IN 46208
(317) 283-6352

Central Ohio Radio Reading Service
229 South High Street
Columbus, OH 43215
(614) 464-2614

Central Piedmont Community College Radio Reading Service
P.O. Box 35009
Charlotte, NC 28235
(704) 342-6994

Central Savannah River Area Radio
Reading Service, Inc.
c/o WACG-FM, Augusta College
2500 Walton Way
Augusta, Georgia 39010
(404) 828-7302

Chicagoland Radio Information Service, Inc.
77 East Randolph Street
Pedestrian Walkway
Chicago, IL 60601
(312) 645-9800

Cleveland Radio Reading Service
1909 East 101st Street
Cleveland, OH 44106
(216) 791-8118

Coastal Area Radio Reading Service, Inc.
701-A Abercorn Street
Savannah, GA 31401
(912) 234-4848

Connecticut Radio Information Services
589 Jordan Lane
Wethersfield, CT 06109
(203) 522-8710

Detroit Radio Information Service
for the Print Handicapped
5057 Woodward Avenue, 15th Floor
Detroit, MI 48202
(313) 577-4146

Education and Reading Service
3520 30th Avenue
Kenosha, WI 53141
(414) 552-9483

El Paso Radio Reading Service
100 Dunne Street
El Paso, TX 79905
(915) 532-4495

Evergreen Radio Reading Service
of the Washington Library for the
Blind and Physically Handicapped
821 Lenora Street
Seattle, WA 98129
(206) 464-6930

Georgia Radio Reading Service, Inc.
1589 Peachtree Street
Atlanta, Georgia 30309
(404) 873-3930

Golden Hours, Inc.
7140 S.W. Macadam
Portland, OR 97219-3013
(503) 229-4804

Golden Triangle Radio Information Center
P.O. Box 3663
Pittsburgh, PA 15230
(412) 434-6023

Greater Lehigh Valley Radio Reading Service
for the Print Handicapped
131 East Broad Street
Bethlehem, PA 18018
(215) 866-8049

Here's To You Radio Reading Service
West Virginia Library Commission
Charleston, WV 25305
(304) 348-4061

Houston Taping for the Blind Radio
3935 Essex Lane
Houston, TX 77027
(713) 622-2767

Idaho Radio Reading Service
341 West Washington
Boise, ID 83720
(208) 334-3220

Illinois Radio Reader
59 East Armory
Champaign, IL 61820
(217) 333-6503

INSIGHT
P.O. Drawer 10K
Milwaukee, WI 53201
(414) 475-8389

In-Sight Radio-Division of In-Sight
235 Promenade Street, Suite 301
Providence, RI 02904
(401) 331-0222

In Touch Networks, Inc.
322 West 48th Street
New York, NY 10036
(212) 586-5588

Jersey Shore Radio Reading Services
c/o WBJB-FM Brookdale Community College
Lyncroft, NJ 07738
(201) 842-1827

KBPS Seeing Sound
546 N.E. 12th Avenue
Portland, OR 97232
(503) 280-5828

KCHO-FM Radio Reading Service
c/o California State University
Communications Department
Chico, CA 95929
(916) 895-5896

Los Angeles Radio Information Service
1570 East Colorado Boulevard
Pasadena, CA 91106
(213) 578-7231

Miami Valley Radio Reading Organization
University of Dayton-Roesch Library
300 College Park Avenue
Dayton, OH 45469
(513) 228-3023

Neighborhood News for the Blind
P.O. Box 7405
Winston-Salem, NC 27109
(919) 761-5257

North Eastern Indiana Radio
Reading Service, Inc.
920 Florence Avenue
Fort Wayne, IN 46808
(219) 422-8230

North Texas Radio Reading Service
3001 Bookhout Street
Dallas, TX 75201
(214) 871-7668

Northern Illinois Radio Information Services
WNIU-FM
Northern Illinois University
DeKalb, IL 60115
(815) 753-0212

Ohio Educational Broadcasting
Network Commission
2470 North Star Road
Columbus, OH 43221
(614) 421-1714

Oklahoma Radio Reading Service
1108 N.E. 36th Street
Oklahoma City, OK 73111
(405) 521-3514

Pell Radio Reading Service for the Blind
228 Adams Avenue
Scranton, PA 18503
(717) 342-7613

Radio Information Center for the Blind
Division of Associated Services for the Blind
919 Walnut Street
Philadelphia, PA 19107
(215) 627-0600

Radio Information Service
Wabash Valley College
2200 College Drive
Mt. Carmel, IL 62963
(618) 262-8641 ext. 253

Radio Information Service for Blind
and Handicapped
9500 West Illinois
Route 15
Belleville, IL 62223
(618) 397-6700

Radio Information Service for Blind and Print Handicapped of
West
Central Illinois
Western Illinois University
504 Memorial Hall
Macomb, IL 61455
(309) 298-2403

Radio Reading Service
P.O. Box 8089
Roanoke, VA 24014
(703) 982-7284

Radio Reading Service for the Blind
Iowa Commission for the Blind
524 Fourth Street
Des Moines, IA 50309
(515) 281-7999

Radio Reading Service of the Association
for the Blind and Handicapped
1912 Eighth Avenue
Altoona, PA 16602
(814) 944-2021

Radio Reading Services, Inc.
817B. Brooklyn Street
Raleigh, NC 27605
(919) 832-5138

Radio Reading Services of Greater
Cincinnati, Inc.
317 East Fifth Street
Cincinnati, OH 45202
(513) 621-4545

Radio Talking Book Network
Minnesota State Services for the Blind and Visually
Handicapped/Communication
Center
1745 University Avenue West
St. Paul, MN 55104
(612) 642-0503

Radio Talking Book Service, Inc.
620 South 31st Street
Omaha, NE 68131
(402) 556-8176

Radio Talking Library
2402 Cherry Street
Erie, PA 16502
(814) 455-0995

Radio Talking Library
244 North Queen Street
Lancaster, PA 17603
(717) 394-7644

Radio Vision
619 North Street
Middletown, NY 10940
(914) 343-1131

Reader Information Service
5100 Rockhill Road
Kansas City, MO 64110
(816) 276-1549

Reading Radio Service
815 North Walnut
Hutchinson, KS 67501
(316) 665-3555

READ-OUT Radio Reading Service
506 Old Liverpool Avenue
Liverpool, NY 13088
(315) 457-0440

RISE
c/o WMHT-FM
P.O. Box 17
Schenectady, NY 12301
(518) 356-1700

San Diego Radio Information Service
San Diego State University
San Diego, CA 92182-0527
(619) 265-6645

Sight Seer
West Michigan Radio Reading Service
3333 E. Beltline NE Avenue
Grand Rapids, MI 49505
(616) 452-9713

Soundsight
Center for Telecommunications Services
University of Texas at Austin
Austin, TX 78712
(512) 471-1631

South Carolina Educational Radio for the Blind
1430 Confederate Avenue
Columbia, SC 29201
(803) 734-7555

Sun Sounds of KJZZ
3124 East Roosevelt Street
Phoenix, AZ 85008
(602) 231-0500

Talking Information Center
130 Enterprise Drive
P.O. Box 519
Marshfield, MA 02050
(617) 834-4400

Trade Winds Radio Reading Service
1800 East 35th Avenue
Gary, IN 46409
(219) 882-5678

University of Kansas Audio Reader Network
P.O. Box 847
Lawrence, KS 66044
(913) 864-4600

UPDATE Radio Reading Service
Chautauqua-Cattaraugus Library System
106 West Fifth Street
P.O. Box 730
Jamestown, NY 14702-0730
(716) 484-7135

Utah State Radio Reading Service
2150 South 300 West
Salt Lake City, UT 84115
(801) 466-6363

Valley Voice Radio Reading Service
for the Print Handicapped
WMRA-FM
James Madison University
Harrisonburg, VA 22807
(703) 568-6221

Virginia Voice for the Print Handicapped
P.O. Box 15546
401 Azalea Avenue
Richmond, VA 23227
(804) 266-2477

Voice of the Peninsula
P.O. Box 1469
2890 George Washington Memorial Highway
Yorktown, VA 23692
(804) 898-0357

Washington Ear, Inc.
35 University Boulevard East
Silver Spring, MD 20901
(301) 681-6636

WCBU Radio Information Service
1501 W. Bradley
Peoria, IL 61602
(309) 672-8577

West Tennessee Talking Library
1850 Peabody Avenue
Memphis, TN 38104
(901) 725-8833

Western Massachusetts Valley Radio Reading Service, Inc.
108 Baldwin Street
West Springfield, MA 01089
(413) 736-8558

Western Montana Radio Reading Services
924 South Third West
Missoula, MT 59801
(406) 721-1998

Wisconsin Radio Reading Service, Inc.
905 University Avenue, Suite 307
Madison, WI 53715
(608) 255-7730

Wichita Radio Reading Service
1751 North Fairmount
Wichita, KS 67208
(316) 682-9121

WKAR Radio Talking Book
c/o WKAR Radio
Michigan State University
East Lansing, MI 48824-1212
(517) 353-9124

WLRH Public Radio
4701 University Drive N.W.
Huntsville, AL 35899
(205) 895-9574

WLRN-FM School Board of Dade County Florida
172 N.E. 15th Street
Miami, FL 33132
(305) 350-3920

WPLN Talking Library
700 Second Avenue
Nashville, TN 37210
(615) 259-5081

WRBH-FM/Radio for the Blind
and Print Handicapped, Inc.
5926 South Front Street
New Orleans, LA 70115
(504) 899-1144

WRKC-Radio Home Visitor
Kings College
Wilkes-Barre, PA 18711
(717) 826-5900

WSFP Radio Reading Service
The University of South Florida
AOC 103
Tampa, FL 33620
(813) 974-4193

WSSR-FM Print Handicapped Service
Sangamon State University
Springfield, IL 62794-9243
(217) 786-6516

WUSF Radio Reading Service
The University of South Florida
AOC 103
Tampa, FL 33620
(813) 974-4193

York County Blind Center's Radio
Reading Service
800 East King Street
York, PA 17403
(717) 848-1690

Appendix I
Rehabilitation Services

Alabama Division of Vocational Rehabilitation
and Crippled Children Service
2129 East South Boulevard
Montgomery, AL 36111-0586

Alaska Office of Vocational Rehabilitation
P.O. Box F
Mail Stop 0581
Juneau, AK 99811-0500
(907) 465-2814

Arizona State Services for the Blind
and Visually Impaired
4620 North 16th Street, Suite 100
Phoenix, AZ 85016
(602) 255-1850 or
Toll-free in Arizona (800) 255-1850

Arkansas Division of Services for the Blind
411 Victory Street
Little Rock, AR 72203
(501) 371-1501 or (501) 371-2587

California Department of Rehabilitation
Central Office
830 K Street Mall
Sacramento, CA 95814
(916) 45-3971 voice
or TDD (telecommunication device for the deaf)

Connecticut State Board of Education
and Services for the Blind
170 Ridge Road
Wethersfield, CT 06109
(203) 249-8525

Delaware Division for the Visually Impaired
305 West Eighth Street
Wilmington, DE 19801
(302) 571-3333

District of Columbia Rehabilitation
Services Administration
Visual Impairment Section
605 G Street, Room 901
Washington, DC 20001
(202) 727-0907

Division of Blind Services
Florida Department of Education
2540 Executive Center West
Tallahassee, FL 32301
(904) 488-1330

Division of Rehabilitation
Colorado Rehabilitation Services
1575 Sherman Street
Denver, CO 80203-4390
(303) 866-4390

Division of Service to the Visually Impaired
South Dakota Department of Vocational Rehabilitation
700 Governors Drive
Pierre, SD 57501
(605) 773-3195

Division of Vocational Rehabilitation
Virgin Islands Department of Social Welfare
P.O. Box 550
Charlotte Amalie
St. Thomas, VI 00801
(809) 774-0930

Division of Vocational Rehabilitation
Wyoming Department of Health
and Social Services
Hathaway Building
2300 Capitol Avenue
Cheyenne, WY 82002
(307) 777-7385

Georgia Division of Rehabilitation Services
878 Peachtree Street, N.E.
Atlanta, GA 30309
(404) 894-6670

Guam Department of Vocational Rehabilitation
GCIC Building, 9th Floor
414 West Soledad Avenue
Agana, GU 96910
011+(671) 472-8806

Hawaii Department of Human Services
Services for the Blind Branch
1901 Bachelot Street
Honolulu, HI 96817
(808) 548-7408

Idaho Commission for the Blind
341 West Washington
Boise, ID 83720
(208) 334-3220

Illinois Department of Rehabilitation Services
General Administration
622 Washington Street
Springfield, IL 62701
(217) 782-2093

Indiana Rehabilitation Services
Division of Services for the Blind
and Visually Impaired
251 North Illinois Street
P.O. Box 7083
Indianapolis, IN 46207-7083
(317) 232-1433

Iowa Commission for the Blind
524 Fourth Street
Des Moines, IA 50309
(515) 281-7999 or Toll-free in Iowa (800) 362-2587

Kansas Division of Services for the Blind
Biddle Building
2700 West Sixth Street
Topeka, KS 66606
(913) 296-4454

Kentucky Department for the Blind
427 Versailles Road
Frankfort, KY 40601
(502) 564-4754

Louisiana Division of Blind Services
Department of Social Services
8225 Florida Boulevard
P.O. Box 94371
Baton Rouge, LA 70804–9371
(504) 342-5284

Maine Bureau of Rehabilitation
Division of Eye Care
32 Winthrop Street
Augusta, ME 04330
(207) 289-3484

Maryland Division of Vocational Rehabilitation
200 West Baltimore Street
Baltimore, MD 21201
(301) 659-2274

Massachusetts State Commission for the Blind
88 Kingston Street
Boston, MA 02111
(617) 727-5550

Michigan Commission for the Blind
Department of Labor
309 North Washington
P.O. Box 30015
Lansing, MI 48909
(517) 373-2062

Minnesota State Services for the Blind
and Visually Handicapped
1745 University Avenue West
St. Paul, MN 55104
(612) 642-0508

Mississippi Vocational Rehabilitation
for the Blind
P.O. Box 4872
5455 Executive Place
Jackson, MS 39216-0872
(601) 354-6411

Missouri Bureau for the Blind
619 East Capital Avenue
Jefferson City, MO 65103
(314) 751-4249

Nebraska Division of Rehabilitation Services
for the Visually Impaired
4600 Valley Road
Lincoln, NE 68510
(402) 471-2891

Nevada Bureau of Services to the Blind
Kinkead Building
505 East King Street, Room 503
Carson City, NV 89710
(702) 885-4444

New Hampshire Division of Vocational Rehabilitation
Bureau of Blind Services
78 Regional Drive
Building JB
Concord, NH 03301
(603) 271-3537

New Jersey Commission for the Blind and Visually Impaired
1100 Raymond Boulevard
Newark, NJ 07102
(201) 648-3333 or
Toll-free in New Jersey (800) 962-1233
(including TDD, telecommunication device
for the deaf)

New Mexico Commission for the Blind
Pera Building, Room 205
Santa Fe, NM 87502
(505) 982-4555

New York State Commission for the Blind
and Visually Handicapped
40 North Pearl Street
Albany, NY 12243
(518) 474-6812

North Carolina Department of Human Resources
Division of Services for the Blind
309 Ashe Avenue
Raleigh, NC 27606
(919) 733-9822

North Dakota Office of Vocational Rehabilitation
Capitol Building
Bismarck, ND 58505
(701) 224-2907

Ohio Rehabilitation Services Commission
Bureau of Services for the Visually Impaired
400 East Campus-View Boulevard
Columbus, OH 43235-4604
(614) 438-1255

Oklahoma State Office of Visual Services
2409 North Kelly Street
Oklahoma City, OK 73126
(405) 424-6006

Oregon State Commission for the Blind
535 S.E. 12th Avenue
Portland, OR 97214
(503) 238-8375

Pennsylvania Bureau of Blindness
and Visual Services
P.O. Box 2675
Harrisburg, PA 17105
(717) 787-6176 or
Toll-free in Pennsylvania (800) 622-2892

Rhode Island Services for the Blind
and Visually Impaired
27 Westminster Street
Providence, RI 02903
(401) 277-2300

South Carolina Commission for the Blind
1430 Confederate Avenue
Columbia, SC 29201
(803) 734-7522 or
Toll free in South Carolina (800) 922-2222

Tennessee Division of Rehabilitation Services
Citizens Plaza Building, 11th Floor
400 Deaderick Street
Nashville, TN 37219
(615) 741-2095

Texas Commission for the Blind
Administration Building
P.O. Box 12866
Austin, TX 78711
(512) 459-2500

Utah Division of Services
for the Visually Handicapped
309 East First South
Salt Lake City, UT 84111
(801) 533-9393

Vermont Division for the Blind
and Visually Impaired
Osgood Building
103 South Main Street
Waterbury, VT 05676
(802) 241-2210

Virginia Department
for the Visually Handicapped
397 Azalea Avenue
Richmond, VA 23227
(804) 371-3140

Visual Services Division
Montana Department of Social
and Rehabilitation Services
111 Sanders
P.O. Box 4210
Helena, MT 59604
(406) 444-2590

Vocational Rehabilitation Program
Puerto Rico Department of Social Services
Box 1118
Hato Rey, PR 00919
(809) 725-1792 or (809) 724-7400, ext. 2335

Washington State Department
of Services for the Blind
921 Lakeridge Drive
Room 202, Mail Stop FW-21
Olympia, WA 98504-2921
(206) 586-1224

West Virginia Division
of Vocational Rehabilitation
State Capitol Building
Charleston, WV 25305
(304) 766-4600

Wisconsin Division of Vocational
Rehabilitation Services for the Blind
P.O. Box 7852
1 West Wilson Street
Madison, WI 53707
(608) 266-1281

Appendix J
Sports and Recreation Organizations and Publications

Access to Art: An Art Resource Directory
for the Blind and Visually Impaired
American Foundation for the Blind
15 West 16th Street
New York, NY 10011
(212) 620-2000

American Alliance for Health Physical Education and
Recreation for the
Handicapped
Information and Research Utilization Center
1201 16th Street, N.W.
Washington, DC 20036
(202) 833-5547

American Alliance for Health, Physical Education, Recreation
and Dance
1900 Association Drive
Reston, VA 22091
(703) 476-3481

American Blind Bowling Association
150 N. Bellair Avenue
Louisville, KY 40206
(502) 896-8039

American Blind Bowling Association
3500 Terry Drive
Norfolk, VA 23518
(804) 857-7267

American Blind Golfers Association
300 Carondelet Street
New Orleans, LA 70112

American Blind Skiing Foundation
610 S William Street
Mt. Prospect, IL 60056
(312) 253-4292 or (312) 255-1739

American Camping Association
Bradford Woods
Martinsville, IN 46151
(317) 342-8456

American National Red Cross
Program of Swimming for the Handicapped
17th and D Streets, N.W.
Washington, DC 20006
(202) 857-3542

Association of Handicapped Artists
1034 Rand Building
Buffalo, NY 14203
(716) 842-1010

Bibles and Other Scriptures in Special Media
National Library Service for the Blind and Physically
Handicapped
Reference Circular
Library of Congress
Washington, DC 20542
(212) 287-5100

Blind Outdoor Leisure Development (BOLD)
533 East Main Street
Aspen, CO 81611
(303) 925-8922

Braille Sports Foundation
7525 North Street
Minneapolis, MN 55426
(612) 935-0423

Choice Magazine
85 Channel Drive
P.O. Box 10
Port Washington, NY 11050
(516) 883-8280

Council for Disabled Sailors
American Sailing Association
13922 Marquesas Way
Marina Del Rey, CA 90290
(213) 822-7171

Dialogue Publications, Inc.
3100 Oak Park Avenue
Berwin, IL 60402
(312) 749-1908

Discovery Blind Sports International
P.O. Box 248
Kirkwood, CA 95646
(209) 258-8600

Evergreen Travel Service
19505 (L) 44 Avenue W
Lynnwood, WA 98036-5699
(206) 776-1184

Hadley School for the Blind
Correspondence Course
700 Elm Street
Winnetka, IL 60093
(312) 446-8111

Handicapped Boaters
P.O. Box 1134, Ansonia Station
New York, NY 10023
(212) 377-0310

Independent Living Aids
11 Commercial Court
Plainview, NY 11803
(516) 752-8080

International Bicycle Tours, Inc.
12 Mid Place
Chappaqua, NY 10514

Kirkwood Instruction for Blind Skiers
P.O. Box 138
Kirkwood, CA 95646

Louis Braille Foundation for Blind Musicians
112 East 19th Street
New York, NY 10003
(212) 627-4646

Matilda Ziegler Magazine
15 West 16th Street
New York, NY 10011
(212) 620-2078

Mobility Tours
26 Court Street, Suite 1110
Brooklyn, NY 11242
(718) 858-6021

National Arts and the Handicapped
Information Service
Arts and Special Constituency Project
National Endowment for the Arts
2401 E Street, N.W.
Washington, DC 20506

National Association of Sports
for Cerebral Palsy
United Cerebral Palsy Association of Connecticut
One State Street
New Haven, CT 06511
(203) 772-2080

National Beep Baseball Association
2421 N. Bell Avenue, Apt. 102
Denton, TX 76201

National Camp Directory for the Blind
and Visually Impaired (In Press)
American Foundation for the Blind
15 West 16th Street
New York, NY 10011
(212) 620-2000

National Committee/Arts for the
Handicapped (NCAH)
1701 K Street, N.W., Suite 801
Washington, DC 20006

National Council for Therapy
and Rehabilitation through Horticulture
9041 Comprint Court, Suite 103
Gaithersburg, MD 20877
(301) 948-3010

National Exhibits by Blind Artists
919 Walnut Street, First Floor
Philadelphia, PA 19107

National Gardening Association
180 Flynn Avenue
Burlington, VT 05401
(802) 863-1308

National Handicapped Sports
and Recreation Association
1145 19th Street, N.W., Suite 717
Washington, DC 20036
(301) 652-7505

National Library Service for the Blind
and Physically Handicapped
Library of Congress
Washington, DC 20542
(202) 287-5100

National Park Service
Department of the Interior
18th and C Streets, N.W.
Washington, DC 20240
(202) 343-6843

National Therapeutic Recreation Society
1601 N. Kent Street
Arlington, VA 22209
(703) 525-0606

North American Riding Association
P.O. Box 100
Ashburn, VA 22011
(703) 777-3540

North American Riding for the Handicapped Association, Inc.
111 East Wacker Drive, Suite 600
Chicago, IL 60601
(312) 644-6610

Outward Bound
Box 250
Long Lake, MN 55350
(612) 473-5476

The President's Committee on Employment
of the Handicapped
Subcommittee on Recreation and Leisure
Washington, DC 20210

The Riding School, Inc.
275 South Avenue
Weston, MA 02193
(617) 899-4555

Science Products
Box A
Southeastern, PA 19399
(215) 296-2111

S.I.R.E., Inc.
(Self-Improvement through Riding Education)
91 Old Bolton Road
Stow, MA 01775
(617) 897-3396

Skating Association for the Blind
and Handicapped, Inc.
3900 Main Street
c/o Sibley's
Buffalo, NY 14226
(716) 833-2994

Ski for Light
1455 West Lake Street
Minneapolis, MN 55408
(612) 827-3232

Society for the Advancement of Travel
for the Handicapped (SATH)
26 Court Street
Brooklyn, NY 11242
(718) 858-5483

Sports Illustrated (published by Time, Inc.)
Available through National Library Service
for the Blind and Physically Handicapped
1291 Taylor Street, N.W.
Washington, DC 20542

Travel Industry and Disabled Exchange (TIDE)
5435 Donna Avenue
Tarzana, CA 91356

Travel Information Center
Moss Rehabilitation Hospital
12th Street and Tabor Road
Philadelphia, PA 19141

United States Association for Blind Athletes
33 N. Institute Street
Brown Hall, Suite 015
Colorado Springs, CO 80903
(719) 630-0422

United States Association for Blind Athletes
55 West California Avenue
Beach Haven, NJ 08008
(609) 492-1017

United States Association for Blind Athletes Newsletter
33905 Calle Acordarse
San Juan Capistrano, CA 92675

United States Blind Chess Association
30 Snell Street
Brockton, MA 02410

United States Blind Golfers Association
225 Barone Street
New Orleans, LA 70112

Bibliography

ABLEDATA. "Electronic Travel Aids Printout." Newington, Connecticut: ABLEDATA, 1989.

_____. "Kurzweil Reader Printout." Newington, Connecticut: ABLEDATA, 1989.

_____. "Speech Synthesizers Printout." Newington, Connecticut: ABLEDATA, 1989.

_____. "Voice Output Module." Newington, Connecticut: ABLEDATA, 1989.

American Foundation for the Blind. "A Different Way of Seeing." New York: AFB, 1984.

_____. "Aging and Vision." New York: AFB, 1987.

_____. *Directory of Services for Blind and Visually Impaired Persons in the United States*, 23rd ed. New York: AFB, 1988

_____. "A Good Employee Is a Good Employee." New York: AFB, 1987.

_____. "Low Vision Questions and Answers: Definitions, Devices, Services." New York: AFB, 1987.

_____. *A Step-By-Step Guide to Personal Management for Blind Persons.* New York: AFB, 1974.

_____. "Understanding and Living with Glaucoma." New York: AFB 1984.

_____. "What Do You Do When You See a Blind Person?" New York: AFB, 1970.

Arkenstone Inc. "Arkenstone Reader with TrueScan." Sunnyvale, California: Arkenstone, 1989.

Artic Technologies. "Artic Crystal." Troy, Michigan: AT, 1989.

Berkeley Systems Inc. "inLARGE: The Software Magnifying Glass." Berkeley, California: BSI, 1989.

BIT Corporation. "Winter 1989 Catalog, Edition #9." Boston: BIT, 1989.

Brock, Peter. *Love in the Lead*. New York: E.P. Dutton, 1954.

Butler, Beverly. *Maggie By My Side*. New York: Dodd, Mead and Company, 1987.

Clearinghouse on the Handicapped. *Programs for the Handicapped*.Washington, D.C.: CH, 1983

Coombs, Jan. *Living With the Disabled: You Can Help*. New York: Sterling Publishing Co. Inc., 1984

Curtis, Patricia. *Greff: The Story of a Guide Dog*. New York: E.P. Dutton, 1982.

Dickman, Irving R. *Making Life More Livable*. New York: American Foundation for the Blind, 1983.

Dietl, Dick. "Operation Job Match: Helping Fill the Worker Void." Worklife (January/February/March 1988): pp. 10-11.

Eden, John. *The Eye Book*. New York: Penguin Books, 1978.

Enabling Technologies Company. "The Marathon Brail-

ler." Stuart, Florida: ETC, 1989.

Galloway, N.R. *Common Eye Diseases and Their Management*. Berlin: Springer-Verlag, 1985.

Guide Dog Foundation for the Blind Inc. "Guide Dog Foundation for the Blind Inc. Training Program." Smithtown, New York: GDFB, 1989.

Hagen, Dolores. *Microcomputer Resource Book for Special Education*. Reston, Virginia: Reston Publishing Company Inc., 1984.

Hendin, David. *Death as a Fact of Life*. New York: W.W. Norton and Company Inc., 1973.

Henter-Joyce Inc. "The Experts in Access Technology." St Petersburg, Florida: HJI, 1989.

Hoshmand, Lisa T. "Blindisms: Some Observations and Propositions." Education of the Visually Handicapped (May 1975): pp. 56-59.

HumanWare Inc. "Braille-n-Print." Loomis, California: HWI, 1989.

IBM Corporation. *Resource Guide for Persons with Vision Impairments*. Atlanta: IBM, 1989.

Jackson, Tom, and Paul Krantz. "Removing Everyday Barriers." Better Homes and Gardens (September 1988): pp. 37-41.

Job Accommodation Network. "JAN." Morgantown, West Virginia: JAN, 1989.

John-Hall, Annette. "Blindness Can't Stop These Athletes." San Jose Mercury News, July 14, 1989, pp. 1D.

Koestler, Frances A. *The Unseen Minority*. New York: David McKay Company Inc., 1976.

Kreisler, Nancy, and Jack. *Catalog of Aids for the Disabled*. New York: McGraw Hill, 1982.

Kubler-Ross, Elisabeth. *On Death and Dying*. New York: Macmillan Publishing Co. Inc., 1969.

_____. *Questions and Answers on Death and Dying*. New York: Macmillan Publishing Co. Inc., 1974.

_____. *Working It Through*. New York: Macmillan Publishing Co. Inc., 1982.

Lauer, Harvey, and Leonard Mowinski. *Computer Aids for the Visually Impaired*. HealthNet Reference Library. Columbus: Compuserve, 1989.

Leflar, Robert B., and Helen Lillie. *Cataracts*. Washington, D.C.: Public Citizen's Health Research Group, 1981.

Ludwig, Irene, Lynne Luxton, and Marie Attmore. *Creative Recreation for Blind and Visually Impaired Adults*. New York: American Foundation for the Blind, 1988.

Mueller, Conrad G., and Mae Rudolph. *Light and Vision*. New York: David McKay Company Inc., 1976.

National Association for Visually Handicapped. "Every Low Vision Patient Should Know..." New York: NAVH, 1985.

_____. "Fact Sheet." New York: NAVH, 1985.

National Federation of the Blind. "Do You Know a Blind Person?" New York: NFB, 1988.

_____. *The Post-Secondary Education and Career Development: A Resource Guide for the Blind and Visually Impaired and Physically Handicapped*. Baltimore: NFB, 1981

_____. "What is the National Federation of the Blind?" New York: NFB, 1988.

National Society to Prevent Blindness. "Facts and Figures: Adult Eye Problems." New York: NSPB, 1980.

Northern California Society to Prevent Blindness. *Coping with Sight Loss in Northern California*. San Francisco: NCSPB, 1989.

Peninsula Center for the Blind. *The First Steps*. Palo Alto, California: PCB, 1980.

Raised Dot Computing Inc. "Raised Dot Computing." Madison, Wisconsin: RDC, 1989.

Recording for the Blind. "Recording for the Blind: A Service to People." Princeton, New Jersey: RB, 1986.

Resnick, Rose. *Sun and Shadow*. New York: Atheneum, 1975.

Retinitis Pigmentosa Foundation Fighting Blindness. "Answers to Your Questions About Retinitis Pigmentosa." Baltimore: RPFFB, 1983.

_____. "Night Vision Aid Fact Sheet." Baltimore: RPFFB, 1987.

Reynolds, James D. "Eye Care Professionals." HealthNet Reference Library. Columbus: Compuserve, 1989.

Sardegna, Jill. *The Encyclopedia of Blindness and Vision Impairment*. New York: Facts on File Publications, 1991.

Scholl, Geraldine T. *Foundations of Education for Blind and Visually Handicapped Children and Youth*. New York: American Foundation for the Blind Inc., 1986.

Schroeder, Ruth, and Doris M. Willabee. *Suggestions for the Blind Cook*. Baltimore: National Federation for the Blind.

Seeing Eye Inc. "Q and A: Facts About the Seeing Eye." Morristown, New Jersey: SEI, 1980.

Seeing Technologies Inc. "The SEETEC Systems." Minneapolis: STI, 1989.

Sloane, Louise L. *Recommended Aids for the Partially Sighted*. New York: National Society for the Prevention of Blindness Inc., 1971.

Sullivan, Tom. *If You Could See What I Hear*. New York: Harper Row, 1975.

Talking Computers Inc. "NEWSBITS." Falls Church, Virginia: TCI, 1989.

Telesensory Systems, Inc. "Focus on Technology." Mountain View, California: TSI, 1989.

United States Association for Blind Athletes, "Sports-Scoop: July and August 1989." Colorado Springs: USABA, 1989.

Zinn, Walter J. and Herbert Solomon. *The Complete Guide to Eye Care, Eyeglasses, and Contact Lenses*. Hollywood, Florida: Frederick Fell Publishers Inc., 1986.

Index